Candida Albicans:

The Quiet Epidemic

Stanley Weinberger, C.M.T.

CANDIDA ALBICANS:
THE QUIET EPIDEMIC

Written & Compiled by
Stanley Weinberger,
CERTIFIED METABOLIC TECHNICIAN

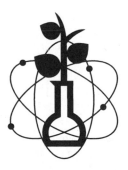

Healing Within Products
San Anselmo, California

01 00 99 98 97 96   5 4 3 2

ISBN 0-9616184-6-9

Edited by Beth Kuper
Cover design & book typography by Allen M. Crider
Proofreading by Margaret Dodd

Question:
what about coffee bean / cigarette token factor?

Contents

PRODUCT DESCRIPTIONS

Candida Albicans Overgrowth

by William Wolcott

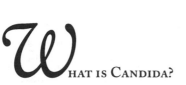

WHAT IS CANDIDA?

Candida albicans is a yeast that lives in the mouth, throat, intestines, and genitourinary tract of most humans. Candida is usually considered to be a normal part of the bowel flora (the organisms that coexist in our lower digestive tract). A healthy immune system normally keeps candida under control, but when the immune system is weakened, the natural balance between the human host and the candida is altered. Unless the body's defenses are given some assistance, colonies of candida will flourish throughout the body producing many adverse physical and mental symptoms collectively known as candidiasis.

We all live in a virtual sea of microorganisms—bacteria, viruses, fungi, and so forth. These microbes can reside in the throat, mouth, nose, intestinal tract, or almost anywhere; they are as much a part of our bodies as the food we eat. Usually, these microorganisms do not cause illness, unless our resistance becomes lowered.

Candida is actually a member of a broader classification of organisms known as fungi. Traditionally, fungi are considered plants, but they contain no chlorophyll and cannot make their own food. Fungi are found in the air we breathe as well as in moist,

I

shady soil, water, manure, dead leaves, fruit, leftover food, and in a wide variety of places and circumstances.

How Do You Get Candida?

Candida albicans prefers people. Candida enters newborn infants during or shortly after birth. Usually, the growth of the yeast is kept in check by the infant's immune system and thus produces no overt symptoms. But, should the immune response weaken, conditions known as oral thrush and diaper rash can result. By six months of age, 90 percent of all babies test positive for candida. And by adulthood, virtually all humans play host to *Candida albicans* and are thus engaged in a lifelong relationship.

Three primary factors weaken the immune system and promote the abnormal growth of candida in the body: 1) poor dietary habits, especially excessive intakes of sugars, starches, yeast-containing products, and processed food; 2) repeated use of antibiotics; 3) the use of hormonal medications such as corticosteroids and birth control pills; and 4) protozoa and other parasitic infestations.

Candida coexists in our bodies with many species of bacteria in a competitive balance. Other bacteria act in part to keep candida growth in check, unless that balance is upset. In a healthy person, the the immune system keeps candida proliferation under control, but when immune response is weakened, candida growth can proceed unhindered. Candida is an "opportunistic organism" which, when given the opportunity, will attempt to colonize all bodily tissues. The uncontrolled growth of candida is known as candida overgrowth.

Do You Have Candida?
- Do you have digestive problems such as indigestion, constipation, diarrhea, bloating, or gas?
- Have you, at any time in your life, taken antibiotics for acne, respiratory, urinary, or other infections?
- Have you taken corticosteroids or immunosuppressive drugs?
- Do you have a preference for sweets, breads, or alcoholic drinks?

- Are you bothered by athlete's foot, psoriasis, or other chronic fungal infestations of the skin?
- Have you ever been diagnosed with parasites?
- Have you ever been troubled with diarrhea or other intestinal problems when traveling?
- Do you experience fatigue, depression, poor memory, or nervous tension?
- Have you even been troubled by persistent prostatitis or vaginitis?
- Do you feel bad all over and no one has been able to determine why?

If you answered yes to three or more of the above questions, candida overgrowth may play a role in causing your symptoms.

CAUSES OF CANDIDA OVERGROWTH

It is well known that the immune system is highly dependent on the proper biochemical balance in the body. Unfortunately, there are many factors in our modern society that can upset the ecological balance of the body, weaken the immune system, and thus allow yeast to overgrow. Many physicians cognizant of candida report that 50 to 70 percent of their patients have candida overgrowth. These seemingly epidemic proportions are attributed to the general decline of vitality—specifically in relation to the immune system—in our society as a result of generations of suboptimal diets and other associated factors of drug and chemical exposure.

Traditional foods have been notably replaced by severely altered foods from a multitude of "modern" treatment methods in growing, processing, and packaging. Heating, pressurizing, preserving, refining, stabilizing, and even creating synthetic foods have all resulted in the considerable alteration of nutrient intake from what had been the previous norm for thousands of years.

Radical alterations in life-style that have accompanied rapid modernization in the twentieth century have brought unforseen and previously uncommon stresses that the human body must now cope with in its efforts at adaptation. Pollution of our air, water, and food; new medications and drugs, both prescription and nonprescription; alcohol; tobacco; high carbohydrate and sugar intake in our diets; chronic food and chemical allergies—all put a considerable strain on the immune system.

There is a growing awareness of the link between major illnesses, such as cancer, diabetes, heart disease, and schizophrenia, to diet and environmental factors and their adverse affects on the immune system. *Candida albicans*, usually a benign yeast held in check by the immune system, proliferates when the immune system becomes unbalanced, compromised, or weakened. The major risk factors that may predispose you to the proliferation of candida are the following:

Antibiotics and Sulfa Drugs. Probably the chief culprit of all, antibiotics kill all bacteria; they do not distinguish the good from the bad. Antibiotics kill the "good" flora that normally keep candida under control. This allows for unchecked growth of candida in the intestinal tract.

It is normally difficult to recover a yeast culture from bodily surfaces. However, after 48 hours of taking tetracycline, yeast can be cultivated easily from anyone. The prevalence today of candida may be most directly related to the widespread societal exposure to antibiotics—from prescriptions for colds, infections, and acne, and from the additional consumption of antibiotic-treated foods, such as meats, dairy, poultry, and eggs.

The rapid and direct proliferation of yeast following antibiotic use strongly suggests that the problem of candida is one that stems from an inner state of imbalance, rather than from an outside attack by a microbe or disease.

Steroid Hormones and Immunosuppressant Drugs. These drugs, such as cortisone, treat severe allergic problems by paralyzing the immune system's ability to react.

Pregnancy, Multiple Pregnancies, or Birth Control Pills. These upset the body's hormonal balance.

Improper Diet. Diets high in carbohydrates, sugar intake, yeast and yeast products, molds, and fermented foods encourage candida overgrowth.

Environmental Hazards. Prolonged exposure to environmental molds as well as an increasing number of chemicals in food, water, and air, including petrochemicals, formaldehyde, perfumes, cleaning fluids, insecticides, tobacco, and other indoor and outdoor pollutants, make the system more susceptible to yeast imbalance.

Once begun, candida overgrowth can result in a self-perpetuating, negative cycle if not recognized and treated appropriately. Large numbers of yeast colonies can weaken the immune system, which normally protects the body from harmful invaders. The immune system may concurrently be adversely affected by poor nutrition and heavy exposure to environmental toxins.

The resulting lowered resistance may not only cause an overall sense of ill health, or the development of respiratory, digestive, and other systemic symptoms. People may also become predisposed to developing sensitivities to foods and chemicals in the environment. Such "allergies" may in turn cause the membranes of the nose, throat, ears, bladder, and intestinal tract to swell and develop infection.

These conditions may lead the physician to prescribe a "broad spectrum" antibiotic that then further promotes the overgrowth of candida and strengthens the existing negative chain of events, leading to further stress on the immune system and increased candida-related problems.

WHAT ARE THE SIGNS OF CANDIDA INFECTIONS?

The result of heightened candida overgrowth is a list of adverse symptoms of considerable length. Basically, the characteristics of candida overgrowth fall under three categories: those affecting the gastrointestinal and genitourinary tracts; allergic responses; and mental/emotional manifestations.

Initially, the signs will show near the sites of original yeast colonies. Most often, the first signs are seen in conditions such as nasal congestion and discharge, nasal itching, blisters in the mouth, sore or dry throat, abdominal pain, belching, bloating, heartburn, constipation, diarrhea, rectal burning or itching, vaginal discharge, vaginal itching or burning, increasingly worsening symptoms of PMS (premenstrual syndrome), prostatitis, impotence, frequent urination, burning on urination, and bladder infections.

But, if the immune system remains weak long enough, candida can spread to all parts of the body causing an additional plethora of problems. Most commonly these include the gastrointestinal tract with all manner of digestive disturbances, food allergies, sensitivities, and cravings for sweets; central nervous system disorders, such as fatigue, drowsiness, incoordination, lack of concentration, dizziness, headaches; musculoskeletal problems involving joint swelling, migrating aches and pains, and arthritis; hormonal disruptions, such as menstrual irregularities; problems with eyes, ears, and the respiratory system, such as spots in front of the eyes, failing vision, burning or tearing eyes, ear pain and deafness, bad breath, coughing, wheezing, asthma, and hay fever; skin problems, such as hives, rashes, eczema, psoriasis, dry skin, and chronic fungal infections, such as athlete's foot, ringworm, and fingernail/toenail infections; impairment of the circulatory system, such as cold hands and feet, numbness and tingling sensations; and aberrations in personality and behavior, such as anxiety, depression, hyperirritability, and mood swings.

In addition, 79 different toxic products are known to be released by candida, which places a considerable burden on the immune system. These toxins get into the bloodstream and travel to all parts of the body where they may cause a host of adverse symptoms.

In candida overgrowth, the yeast colonies can dig deep into intestinal walls, damaging the bowel wall. Candida can also attack the immune system, causing supressor cell disease, in which the immune system produces antibodies to everything at the slightest provocation, resulting in extreme sensitivities. Finally, candida overgrowth can be dangerous if not controlled. The persistent, constant challenge to the immune system by an ever-increasing, long-term overgrowth of candida can eventually serve to wear down the immune system and cause a seriously weakened capacity for resistance to disease.

Women are more likely to get candida overgrowth than are men. This is related to the female sex hormone progesterone, which is elevated in the last half of the menstrual cycle. Progesterone increases the amount of glycogen (animal starch, easily converted to sugar) in the vaginal tissues, which provides an ideal growth medium for candida. Progesterone levels also elevate during pregnancy. Men are affected less frequently but are by no means invulnerable.

HOW DO YOU KNOW YOU HAVE CANDIDA?

Currently, diagnosis is primarily clinical. Since almost all people have candida in their bodies, tests for its presence are useless; confirmation of overgrowth is very difficult through laboratory tests. And, since candida paralyzes the immune system, allergy tests to determine the system's reaction to it are also ineffectual.

Furthermore, the results of the yeast imbalance—the combined effects of different hormones, poisons generated and released by the yeast into the bloodstream, and the confusion created in the immune system—produce a wide variety of symptoms that are seemingly unrelated (such as wheezing, depression, and fungus infection under fingernails). Thus, it is difficult to make a definite diagnosis from any specific pattern of signs and symptoms.

Currently, the best test still seems to be the therapeutic trial. A joint decision is usually made by the physician and the patient after analyzing the individual's case history. (Many physicians regard vaginal yeast infections as the most reliable indicator of candida overgrowth in women, for example.) A tentative diagnosis is made, based on the patient's history of symptoms in relation to any known possible predisposing factors, which is then proven true or false by the way the patient responds to therapy.

Many physicians now believe that a clinical trial for candida overgrowth is of so little risk or expense that it should be considered in any chronic illness. One clinical trial you may try for five days is to avoid eating certain foods that are known to facilitate the growth of yeast. Such foods include the following:

Sugar and Carbohydrates found in all sweetened foods, including honey, molasses, sorghum, maple syrup, sugar, fructose, maltose, and dextrose. Also, fresh fruits, dried fruits, and fresh, frozen, and canned juices should be eliminated, as well as soda pop.

Yeast Products, such as beer, wine, sake, liquor, bread, natural B vitamins, and brewer's yeast.

Fermented and Mold Foods, such as mushrooms, cheese, vinegar, mustard, catsup, relish and other condiments made with vinegar, sour cream, buttermilk, tofu, soy sauce, and miso.

After eliminating these foods for five days, try adding them back into your diet in large quantities. By observing how you feel while off these foods, in comparison to any adverse affects experienced when going back on the foods, you may get a clue as to any possible yeast involvement as a causative factor for any adverse symptoms.

How Do You Reduce Candida Overgrowth?

Although diagnosis and supervision of treatment requires a physician, the reacquisition of health and control of candida by the immune system also depends a great deal on the effort of the candida patient. Generally, treatment of candida involves four major considerations:

1. Destroying the yeast.
2. Eliminating, if possible, immunosuppressive drugs and antibiotics, or curtailing their use to only when absolutely necessary.
3. Depriving the candida of those foods on which it is nourished and flourishes.
4. Rebalancing and strengthening of the body's immune system for the restoration of proper function through dietary measures that will meet individual nutritional requirements.

To destroy candida, or "to even the odds" so to speak, a physician may prescribe a drug by the name of nystatin, or one of several available products containing nystatin. It is an antibiotic, which means that it is made by one kind of germ, such as a mold, to kill another germ, such as strep, staph, or tuberculosis.

Nystatin is an antibiotic that kills yeasts and only yeasts. It is one of the least toxic known drugs; even when large amounts are ingested, only small traces actually get into the bloodstream. The pure powdered form is generally accepted as most effective.

Nystatin and caprylic acid products are deadly to candida. Depending on the severity of candida overgrowth and the amount of the agents taken, the candida can be killed off in vast numbers in a very short period of time. As they are killed, they release substances that are toxic to the body. If this process occurs more quickly than the toxins can be cleared from the bloodstream and eliminated by the body, a temporary toxic or allergic-type reaction can occur. The technical name for this experience is a "Herxheimer reaction," more commonly referred to as "die-off."

Usually die-off lasts only a few hours, although it can last several days. It can usually be controlled almost entirely by the amount of ingestion of the agent and the rate or frequency it is taken. Signs of Herxheimer reaction can be many and varied, but generally involve such discomfort as aching, bloating, nausea, and an overall "goopy sick" feeling, or a worsening of original symptoms. Fortunately, die-off is generally short in duration, and although uncomfortable, is at least a confirmation of the presence of candida and that something good is happening.

Exercise, colonics, and enemas are helpful in countering the adversities of die-off.

Although nystatin is very effective in killing candida, many people develop an allergic-type sensitivity to it with prolonged use. For this reason, many physicians are now considering alternatives for the job. Foremost among these is the use of products containing caprylic acid.

Caprylic acid is a natural substance, a fatty acid, that is totally lethal to candida. It is available over the counter and appears to be equal to nystatin in effectiveness, and is not known to produce the sensitivity side effects of nystatin. Of the caprylic acid products on the market, Caprystatin, Kaprycidin-A, and Orithrush-D Gargle, when used together, appear to be the most effective by virtue of their capacity to address the entire digestive tract.

Other natural aids in the fight against candida are garlic and Pau D'Arco (or Taheebo) tea, both believed to have natural fungicidal properties. Garlic is preferably taken raw, but may be effectively utilized in capsule form in a product called Arizona Natural Garlic.

Proper Diet

Research has found that the immune system is highly sensitive to the proper biochemical balance in the body, which affects the immune system's efficient functioning. A growing amount of nutritional research suggests that although everyone requires the same nutrients to maintain metabolic processes, different people need different amounts of nutrients to meet optimal requirements of their nutritional individuality.

For these reasons, Healthexcel provides a scientific means of identifying nutritional requirements based on the determination of the individual's "metabolic type," i.e., the genetically determined metabolic and nutritional parameters. It is because different people have different metabolic types, and therefore different needs for nutrition, that the allopathic, symptom-treatment approach in nutrition is baseless and so often ineffective. This further explains why, nutritionally, what helps make one person feel better may have little or no effect on another, or even make a third person feel worse. Once the metabolic type is determined, a diet and supplementation program can be recommended to meet individual nutrition requirements, thus providing an ideal means of restoring proper biochemical balance.

In addition, the use of natural, live acidophilus culture, such as that found in the product DDS, has been found helpful in aiding the body to restore the proper intestinal flora balance.

Many people with candida overgrowth find it very difficult to "get off" an antifungal agent, such as nystatin or caprylic acid, without a recurrence of the problem. In lieu of such circumstances, consider the following:

- If different people have different requirements for nutrition; and
- If the immune system is highly dependent on the proper bio-chemical balance to function efficiently; and
- If the immune system is supposed to keep candida in check; and
- If the problem of candida overgrowth recurs when you stop the antifungal agent, then it is possible that you are following a diet that is inappropriate for your immune system, which may in part be responsible for your body's failure to control the yeast.

Ideally, then, it is HEALTHEXCEL's recommendation that the attending physician suggest that anyone with candida overgrowth adhere to a diet that is correct for that person's metabolic type.

Unfortunately, it's not sufficient to get rid of the symptoms of candida overgrowth to the exclusion of the underlying cause of the problem—a compromised immune system. Thus, if you ignore your nutritional individuality, you may also find that although you are temporarily successful in ridding your system of candida, your success may be short-lived and you may experience a recurrence of the problem. The next logical step is to improve your overall immune efficiency by addressing your individual metabolic requirements.

CONCLUSION

Total elimination of yeast from the body is neither feasible nor desirable, considering that yeasts are very likely beneficial to the body when a proper balance exists. Treatment of candida overgrowth does not seek the eradication of candida from the person, but rather a *restoration of the proper and bal-*

anced relationship between the person and the yeast.

Candida albicans, if uncontrolled, may indeed pose a serious threat to health and well-being. Another perspective, however, may view candida as a kind of "early warning system." Candida in a well-balanced body chemistry is merely a part of a greater environmental whole that provides some benefit to the host with whom it coexists.

It is only when the body chemistry becomes imbalanced and the immune system is compromised as a result that overgrowth becomes a problem to be reckoned with. It is a signal to us that drugs, improper foods, or other forms of distress have significantly weakened our defenses and undermined our good health. Viewed from this perspective, the presence of early warning signals afforded us by *Candida albicans* may actually allow for the avoidance of future disaster.

How to Fight
Candida and Survive

by Tom Valentine

❧ —— ❧

"*U*ntreated systemic candidiasis has a mortality rate approaching 100 percent. Delay in treatment is dangerous and will almost certainly end in death of the patient."

That telling statement was written by Dr. Richard Hurley of London in a medical paper.

"When tests are done on estrogen levels, thyroid levels, or other hormone levels and people are suffering from these symptoms (candidiasis), the hormones are there in the bloodstream, but they are not activating any response."

Orian Truss, M.D., the leading authority on chronic candidiasis, made the statement above when describing the insidious attacks the common fungus *Candida albicans* makes on the human endocrine and immune systems.

Hormones are essential to our health, and our bloodstream must be literally crawling with them in order for our bodies to operate in a normal, balanced manner. When candidiasis takes hold of the endocrine system and imbalances hormonal function, a major health problem developes that has yet to be fully diagnosed and understood by the mainstream medical establishment.

Candidiasis has a way of disarming our immune systems, and if that sounds like AIDS (Acquired Immune Deficiency Syndrome) to you, join the club that is seeing more links between the two deadly infections than the establishment cares to admit.

There is strong sentiment among Americans that the drug-monopolized, bureaucratically-controlled medical establishment has failed them. More and more people are looking back at their medical histories and seeing that what they had previously suffered was undiagnosed chronic candidiasis.

A NATURAL WAR

There is a war going on inside every one of us. It's a war between natural microbes in our systems, and we have been losing for decades because of our medical establishment's combination of arrogance and ignorance, or criminal neglect, or both.

Our vital endocrine system (thyroid, thymus, parathyroid, pineal, pituitary, adrenal, pancreas, ovaries, testes) should not be infected by naturally occurring intestinal fungus. But, it is—with devastating, generally undiagnosed effects.

The drug industry lock on medical technology and education has helped create an arrogant ignorance within the profession that has been further enhanced by monopolistic bureaucracy. To now be told by courageous researchers, defying established dogma, that the "wonder drugs" of the past have unleashed an epidemic of immune-destroying chronic candidiasis, calls for charges of criminal negligence.

Why do a few independent researchers have to put their reputations on the line and "discover" that the common yeast, *Candida albicans*, is wreaking havoc with our national health? Why didn't the great institutions learn this natural fact decades ago? Hippocrates, the father of medicine, noted the common candida-caused infections of vaginitis and oral thrush more than 1,500 years before the microscope.

However, to point out the flaws and establish blame does not solve the problem. What's done is done. Now people must act to help themselves, and at the same time to force political changes that will result in a revamping of the medical bureaucracy.

The big problem is to stop candidiasis before it stops us.

Candida has the upper hand because millions remain in ignorance and joyously starve their own systems while feeding the fungus.

AIDS—Plus

How bad is it? Let's look at the latest from the AIDS front. Even those who don't know about candida have heard about AIDS. There's no link between the two, you say. One is virally caused, the other is a mold, you say.

Dr. Robert S. Mendelsohn has pointed out that a bulletin from the medical establishment (*FDA Drug Bulletin*) places some forms of candidiasis in a category now called "lesser AIDS."

In his February 1985 newsletter, the doctor who pointed out the flaws in his profession for the benefit of the people wrote:

"The new, expanded definition of AIDS, of course, raises a new set of questions. The government doctors have reassured us that no cases of AIDS have been found in members of families of AIDS victims. However, with their new definition, those old studies become worthless until the families are restudied for these additional diseases.

Perhaps even more importantly, the HTLV-III test, like any other laboratory test, produces not only false-positive results, but false negatives. Therefore, if a person has one of these diseases now listed under the AIDS umbrella, how do the doctors know that, even in the absence of a positive AIDS blood test, the patient does not have AIDS?"

In case you aren't confused enough , the *FDA Drug Bulletin* states: "In addition, idiopathic thrombocytopenia (a blood condition) is probably associated with the HTLV-III-III infection, as are a variety of non-life threatening fungal and bacterial infectious processes..." The doctors call these manifestations lesser AIDS.

So now we have AIDS, ARC (AIDS related complex) and lesser AIDS. When it comes to the causes of AIDS or its symptomatology, do researchers or government doctors really know what they're talking about?

Based on the in-depth research of Dr. Orian Truss, a physician from Birmingham, Alabama, wrote *The Missing Diagnosis*, and is considered the world's top authority on chronic candidiasis— which is much more than a simple yeast infection, even though the same critter is involved.

Dr. Truss has cured patients of debilitating conditions, which had virtually wrecked their lives, by discovering that the patients were not "neurotic," nor did they need "psychiatry" simply because medicine could not correctly diagnose their chronic candidiasis.

CANDIDA ALBICANS

Candida albicans is among the most common yeasts, molds, and fungi. It may be found in every human intestinal tract from the mouth (it is especially fond of dentures) to the anus, and in every vagina. Normally, the fungus is kept under control by friendly bacteria, such as Lactobacillus acidophilus, so it poses no threat to health.

Many times we hear a person say, "Oh, that's only a yeast infection, that's not serious." This is an attitude nurtured by the establishment's attitude. Obviously a wrong attitude.

"The yeast lives in everyone," Dr. Truss told *Acres U.S.A.* "However, when it is stimulated by various factors, especially antibiotics and birth control pills, it may establish a chronic infection known as chronic candidiasis."

What happens, Dr. Truss explained, is that the yeast is not affected by the broad spectrum antibiotics, which kill off the friendly bacteria by the billions. Antibiotics are the worst, but not the only, drug-induced cause for chronic candidiasis. With the friendly bacteria obliterated, the fungus overgrows its normalcy and the individual's immune system must deal with the spreading mold. "Once candida gets into other tissues and into the bloodstream, it has the ability to overcome the immune system."

That sounds a lot like AIDS, does it not?

To make matters worse, researchers at the University of Iowa discovered that *Candida albicans* has chameleon-like abilities to change its form—making it difficult to control.

According to the *Des Moines Register*, December 30, 1985, biologists at the University of Iowa described the common fungus as "a microscopic monster capable of inflicting a wide range of torture" on patients. "Until recently, however, nobody knew candida very well. Now it appears the common yeast is a more terrible creature than anyone suspected—a Dr. Jekyll and Mr. Hyde character capable of changing back to its original form."

Another aspect that sounds like AIDS!

"Dr. David Soll, the University of Iowa biologist who discovered candida's quick-change ability, says it may be what allows the fungus to elude both antibiotics and the body's immune system," the article added.

It is incredible that the wonders of modern medical technology somehow overlooked this fungus until Dr. Truss and others screamed so loudly they could no longer be ignored.

Now, we note, a number of financial grants are finding their way into universities as the drug monopoly scurries to cover its proverbial behind with patentable pharmacology to stop the spread of this common critter that drugs helped unleash in the first place.

In our technological sophistication, arrogant mankind seems to forget that "it isn't wise to fool mother nature."

Among the data from the study was the discovery that a particular drug, ketoconazole, does not work for "immunosuppressed patients." Immunosuppression is curious logic, unless you think you're smarter than nature.

According to Dr. Truss:

"An immunosuppressant drug is a drug that suppresses or weakens the immune defenses of the body. Many symptoms of illness are actually due to the inflammation that results when the white blood cells respond in defense against some injurious or potentially dangerous factor.

Symptoms may be due to the body's defensive response

to a germ, rather than to the germ itself. A sore throat or the inflamed tissues of the nose and throat characteristic of the common cold are familiar examples. Even when the inflammation is not clearly related to an infectious agent, for example rheumatoid arthritis, it is quite likely that most of the symptoms result from the immune response to an as yet undiscovered cause of the disease."

Since inflammation is distressing to patients, the medical profession happily accepted from drug manufacturers a group of drugs designed to suppress the immune system and make the inflammation go away.

"Unfortunately," Dr. Truss added, "it is not possible to suppress just one manifestation of immunity by impairing the entire immune response."

Cortisone-type hormone drugs are the most commonly used immunosuppressants, and Dr. Truss lists them among the major causes of the epidemic spread of chronic candidiasis.

CONTRIBUTING FACTORS

Let's add it all up. Our society is crawling with pollutants that enhance candida and clobber us. Our food is refined, additivized, and chemicalized, and then so loaded with sugars and starch that we feed candida very happily—beer-belly bloat is an obvious "sign" of candidiasis.

There is also the "health food" known as brewer's yeast. Most B vitamins come in brewer's yeast bases, which serves to strengthen candida.

Infants being breastfed, Dr. Truss said, have a strong *Lactobacillus acidophilus* count and candidiasis is not normally seen. But once off the breast, candidiasis shows up in a hurry—as diaper rash.

The critter is chasing us from cradle to grave—gleefully. One doctor noted that "the living human is nothing more than organic matter that needs recycling to *Candida albicans.*"

Antibiotics are everywhere in our society—in meats and poultry, in the hands of every pediatrician, even over-the-counter. Add the technical wonders of cortisone and birth control pills and you have an epidemic.

The symptoms of chronic candidiasis include:

Central nervous system disorders: depression, anxiety, irrational irritability, lethargy, fatigue, agitation, inability to concentrate, memory loss, and headaches, including migraines.

Intestinal disorders: bloating, diarrhea, constipation, heartburn, gastritis, indigestion, and colitis.

Allergic manifestations: severe chemical and food sensitivities, asthma, acne, hives, sinusitis, hay fever, skin rashes, earaches, and possible psoriasis.

In children there is hyperactivity, irritability, learning problems, poor appetite, and erratic sleep patterns as well as the other symptoms. One of the most used, if not the most used, medical techniques today is the ear-tube operation for children.

What can you do to protect yourself?

Doctors are prescribing nystatin and other prescription drugs, but as with all drugs there are drawbacks and side effects. Besides, there is evidence that when the drugs are halted, the yeast comes back with a vengeance. Some herbalists suggest garlic, but doctors say it is ineffective.

There are a number of independent physicians striving to cope with the pandemic, which is still largely unrecognized by the medical establishment. The best way to avoid or overcome chronic candidiasis is by following a careful dietary program, re-establishing the friendly bacteria, and strengthening the immune system.

Nothing fights *Candida albicans*, in all its forms, better than *Lactobacillus acidophilus*, especially the DDS strain developed at the University of Nebraska.

Note: there is order form for the Healing Within Candida Overgrowth Elimination Program on page 113. This time-proven program is highly effective in combating candida.

CANDIDA ALBICANS SELF-TEST

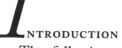

*I*NTRODUCTION

The following questionnaire was designed by William G. Crook, M.D., to be used by adults to identify their predisposition to *Candida albicans* yeast infection. It is not intended as a means for diagnosis, but only as an organized system for gathering information regarding candida. If you score high on this questionnaire, you may wish to bring it to your physician's attention. Your physician may then decide to run clinical tests in order to determine whether or not you have abnormal candida growth presently occurring. Any therapy in this regard will depend on your physician's judgment.

It is not within the jurisdiction of the author to diagnose the presence of candida, nor to recommend any therapeutic action. The author recognizes this activity as the sole responsibility of the attending physician. This material is provided for educational and informational purposes only, in hopes that it may prove of use to you and your physician.

INSTRUCTIONS

Section A pertains to factors in your medical history that may promote the imbalanced growth of candida. Sections B and C are concerned with symptoms commonly seen in individuals with yeast-connected illnesses.

For each "Yes" answer you have in Section A, circle the Point Score in that section. At the end of the section, total your score and record it on the Total Score line. Then move to Sections B and C, and score as indicated.

Section A: History

	Point Score
Have you taken tetracyclines (Sumycin®, Panmycin®, Vibramycin®, Minocin®, etc.) or other antibiotics for acne for one month or longer?	25
Have you at any time in your life taken other "broad-spectrum" antibiotics (ampicillin, amoxicillin, Ceclor®, Bactrim®, Septra®, Keflex®, etc.) for respiratory, urinary, or other infections for two months or longer, or in shorter course, four or more times in a one-year period?	20
Have you taken a broad-spectrum antibiotic drug, even a single course?	6
Have you at any time in your life been bothered by persistent prostatitis, vaginitis, or other problems affecting your reproductive organs?	25

Have you been pregnant:
Two or more times?	5
One time?	3

Have you taken birth control pills:
For more than two years?	15
For two weeks or less?	8

Have you taken prednisone, Decadron®, or other cortisone-type drugs:
For more than two weeks?	15
For two weeks or less?	6

Have you ever been afflicted with a parasitic problem at any time in your life?	20

Does exposure to perfumes, insecticides, fabric shop odors, and other chemicals provoke:

Moderate or severe symptoms?	20
Mild symptoms?	5

Are symptoms worse on damp, muggy days or in moldy places?	20

Have you had athlete's foot, ringworm, jock itch, or other chronic fungus infections of the skin or nails:

Severe or persistent?	20
Mild to moderate?	10
Do you crave sugar?	10
Do you crave breads?	10
Do you crave alcoholic beverages?	10
Does tobacco smoke really bother you?	10

Total Score Section A   _____

SECTION B: MAJOR SYMPTOMS

For each of your symptoms, enter the appropriate figure in the Point Score column:

If a symptom is *occasional or mild*, score 3 points.

If a symptom is *frequent and/or moderately severe*, score 6 points.

If a symptom is *severe and/or disabling*, score 9 points.

	Point Score
Fatigue or lethargy	_____
Feeling of being drained	_____
Poor memory	_____
Feeling spacey or unreal	_____
Depression	_____
Numbness, burning, or tingling	_____
Muscle aches	_____
Muscle weakness or paralysis	_____
Pain and/or swelling in joints	_____
Abdominal pain	_____
Constipation	_____
Diarrhea	_____
Bloating	_____
Troublesome vaginal discharge	_____
Persistent vaginal burning or itching	_____
Prostatitis	_____
Impotence	_____
Loss of sexual desire	_____

Endometriosis _____

Cramps and/or other menstrual irregularities _____

Premenstrual tension (PMS) _____

Spots in front of eyes _____

Erratic vision _____

Total Score Section B _____

Section C: Other Symptoms

For each of your symptoms, enter the appropriate figure in the Point Score column:

If a symptom is *occasional or mild*, score 3 points.

If a symptom is *frequent and/or moderately severe*, score 6 points.

If a symptom is *severe and/or disabling*, score 9 points.

	Point Score
Drowsiness	_____
Irritability or jitteriness	_____
Incoordination	_____
Inability to concentrate	_____
Frequent mood swings	_____
Headaches	_____
Dizziness/loss of balance	_____
Pressure above ears; feeling of head swelling or tingling	_____
Itching	_____
Other rashes	_____
Heartburn	_____
Indigestion	_____
Belching and intestinal gas	_____
Mucous in stools	_____
Hemorrhoids	_____
Dry mouth	_____
Rash or blisters in mouth	_____

Bad breath   _____

Joint swelling or arthritis   _____

Nasal congestion or discharge   _____

Postnasal drip   _____

Nasal twitching   _____

Sore or dry throat   _____

Cough   _____

Pain or tightness in chest   _____

Wheezing or shortness of breath   _____

Urgency or urinary frequency   _____

Burning on urination   _____

Failing vision   _____

Burning or tearing of eyes   _____

Recurrent infections or fluid in ears   _____

Ear pain or deafness   _____

Total Score Section C   _____

Total Score Section A (from page 23)   _____

Total Score Section B (from page 25)   _____

GRAND TOTAL SCORE   _____

SCORING

According to Dr. Crook, yeast-connected health problems are *almost certainly* present in women with scores over 180, and in men with scores over 140. (Women's scores will tend to run higher, as seven items apply exclusively to women, while only two apply exclusively to men.)

Yeast-connected health problems are *probably* present in women with scores over 120, and in men with scores over 90.

Yeast-connected health problems are *possibly* present in women with scores over 60, and in men with scores over 40.

If you feel that you may have a candida overgrowth problem, consider following the HEALING WITHIN 8-Week Candida Overgrowth Elimination Program described on pages 95-104.

OXYGEN THERAPY

$\Longrightarrow$ —— $\Longleftarrow$

*W*HY IT SHOULD BE OF INTEREST TO EVERYONE

For many years the health sciences have been seeking to identify the primary physical cause of all illness and disease, and create a universal remedy that would satisfy the correction of this primary cause. Now both have been found, but their utter simplicity makes them difficult to accept at first.

A toxic digestive system, organ system, and cellular environment is the primary cause of all ailments according to natural principles —not microbes, as we have been led to believe. No one should judge his or her health on the basis of daily evacuations of kidneys or bowels. A person may have regular daily "normal" eliminations, yet still be badly ailing because the assimilation and elimination processes may be unbalanced.

Oxygen Therapy accomplishes the necessary and desired purification of the digestive tract, then purifies every organ, blood vessel, and cell in the entire body. It does this not by burying symptoms as in drug therapy, but by liquefying the waste in the system and passing it out through the bowels and urinary tract.

Growing in the toxic (anaerobic) cellular environment are the microbes (bacteria, viruses, yeast, parasites, etc.) that we hear about so often in medical diagnosis as the main cause of illness or disease. These microbes cannot live in an oxygen-filled (aerobic) environment. You might notice here that Oxygen Therapy not only oxidizes the microbes, thus killing them off, but also eliminates the root cause of their presence in the first place—toxicity in the system.

Oxygen Therapy is an important natural nutritional method for the prevention and elimination of illness and disease. It can be used without interruption of one's work or activities.

Nature demands her time and cannot be hurried. Mild cases of ailments or illness may show splendid results in a few days or weeks, while in more serious cases a marked improvement cannot be expected in so short a time. Nevertheless, the longer the remedy is taken, the more marked the improvement. In more chronic or stubborn so-called incurable diseases, it should not be overlooked that the built-up toxins and medical poisons used to bury symptoms have impaired the metabolism, and cannot be rectified quickly, even by the best of healing methods. Because Oxygen Therapy employs nature's best natural resources and nothing else, its consistent use will not harm, but will give the best possible results.

At the start of Oxygen Therapy, the frequent watery stools, which may appear 3-5 times a day, will cease as soon as your body's system is purified. After that, you may increase your dose if so desired. The released oxygen will follow the blood stream, cleansing the blood vessels and cells. This being the case, we must allow time for the oxygen to reach the extreme parts of the body. Thus, it is impossible to gauge the exact time required for the correction of each case.

The results do not depend on dietary rules, but, of course, far better results are obtained if you refrain from consuming food or drink detrimental to your health. Even a person adhering to an unbalanced diet will feel beneficial results if general rules are consistently followed.

A healing process or reaction (sometimes called a healing crisis) may appear in many cases soon after starting Oxygen Therapy and may reappear at certain intervals in all ailments, especially chronic conditions, until the cause or causes of the ailments are eliminated. This healing process is an act of health which is naturally and nutritionally sound, and no one should become alarmed or discouraged through these natural healing reactions. On the contrary, they should be considered highly welcome as the true signs of a better and healthier future.

Summary

1) A toxic body has to be purified.
2) The damages done by ailments, disease or stress must be repaired.
3) An unhealthy metabolism must be balanced.

These three processes are required to return the body to complete health. Oxygen Therapy goes a long way toward satisfying these requirements for good health. Thousands of people are discovering Oxygen Therapy to be safe and effective against an amazing variety of disorders.

Dr. Joseph LaVolpa, N.D., P.M.D., Ph.D.
Preventive Medicine Specialist
Natural Health Center
Santa Rosa, California

Dear Friends in Health,

What I have to share with you is of such importance that I strongly encourage you to please read through this letter carefully.

Are you experiencing aging problems, lack of energy, ailments, or any kind of physical disorder that is preventing you from enjoying life? Have you tried everything available on the market and given up finding a cure? Please don't despair. There is something you can do, but you may not have heard about it until NOW. I'm talking about OXYGEN THERAPY, and it is available now for the first time in a stabilized powder in capsule form for convenient daily use.

Why oxygen? Here in the 1990s, we are taking in one-half the amount of oxygen of 100 years ago. Since we are an oxygen machine, this lack of oxygen means a significant reduction in our ability to recreate healthy cells. It also means we are creating an internal environment designed for the growth of all kinds of bacteria, viruses, yeasts and toxins. These microbes and toxins cannot exist in an oxygen-filled environment.

It is for this reason that Oxygen Therapy is a breakthrough of staggering and immense importance.

Oxygen Therapy has demonstrated to be a powerful and effective remedy for:

AIDS	Flu
Allergies	Hepatitis
Arthritis	Herpes
Asthma	HIV
Cancer	Metabolic Disorders
Candida Yeast Infection	Parasites
Chronic Fatigue	Reproductive Problems
Circulatory Congestion	Skin Eruptions
Diabetes	Tumors
Digestive Disorders	Urinary Disorders
Epstein-Barr	

I give Oxygen Therapy my strongest endorsement. As a natural doctor, I believe in its capabilities. I know that it works because I've used it with my clients/patients and they report excellent results.

Be young again and live an active physical life free from disease and physical limitation. For the sake of your health and the health of your family, I urge you to try Oxygen Therapy today.

With healthy regards,

Dr. Joseph LaVolpa

Ozone: Its Therapeutic Action

⇛ — ⇚

Ozone (O_3 or O_2O) is an allotropic form of oxygen. It is oxygen in its most active state. It therefore means a more generous supply of oxygen, the life giver and life sustainer.

Through the action of flashes of lightning, nature produces Ozone to purify the air and to destroy all organic decay upon which disease, germs, and bacteria thrive. Like oxygen, Ozone is a healthful gas. It has, however, a much greater oxidizing, antiseptic, and germicidal power, and for this reason it is used with great success for the relief of various diseases. Recently, the FDA and other such suppressive organizations have been trying to negate the beneficial and life-sustaining qualities of Ozone by telling the public that Ozone is poisonous and detrimental to the body. This is not so! For years physicians around the world have used Ozone to bring palliative and curative results to many, many individuals. Famous physicians like Dr. Rokitansky in Vienna, Dr. F. M. Eugene Blass, and others around the world have realized the importance of this tremendous gas.

Ozone is one of the most energetic and useful agents known to science. Its therapeutic action is due to the oxygenation of the blood by the loose molecule (free radical) of oxygen in the O_3 compound. Ozone is carried to the various organs and tissues of the body and absorbed, thus oxidizing waste products and facilitating their elimination. In other words, Ozone increases the metabolism without the expenditure of vital energy. Special stress should be laid on the fact that Ozone is a *natural* remedy.

In the process of respiration, waste products are exposed to the action of the oxygen of the air, and they are burned up very much as if they were put into a stove, thereby producing body heat. In the living body, heat—whether tangible or not—is continually being generated through the chemical action of carbon and oxygen.

When the blood receives sufficient oxygen to unite with carbon, in the proportion of two atoms of oxygen to one of carbon, carbon dioxide or carbonic acid gas (CO_2) is formed, which is in a suitable state to be eliminated. The process of oxidation is complete, the body temperature is maintained at normal (98.6° F), the organs perform their functions properly, and the system is in a condition to resist the toxic influences of microbes, the environment, and mankind's excesses.

When, however, an insufficient amount of oxygen is received by the blood, carbon monoxide is formed (CO), which is NOT readily eliminated, and through its poisonous irritation to the organs, the body temperature is reduced below normal, and system is rendered incapable of resisting the toxic influences of the various bacteria, and environmental and industry related toxins—disease is the result.

So prevalent is subnormal temperature among people who are "rundown," that nine out of ten of them show a subnormal temperature by actual thermometer test. There have been several reasons for subnormal temperatures in recent years. They range from "thyroid insufficiency" to "hypothalamus disorders." These explanations are correct—but only to a degree. The real *cause* of the problem is low and inadequate oxidation or oxygen assimilation. Therefore, the thyroid, hypothalamus, or other endocrine organs (given as the cause) are hindered in their normal metabolic functions, and subnormal temperature is the result. The correct way to counteract this situation is to give a substance that will restore the oxidative process.

The clinical thermometer is the best means of determining the existence of under-oxidation and should be used routinely. The temperature of a person who is under-oxidized run from a fraction to several degrees below normal.

The under-oxidated and subnormal temperatured person will present one or more of the following symptoms: headache, dizziness, insomnia, constipation, feeling faint, loss of appetite, palpitation of the heart, bad kidney action, sporadic and related menstrual problems, cold hands and feet, and various other symptoms, all of which are due to an impoverished blood supply.

From these symptoms, we are justified in rendering an explanation of under-oxidation, taking on the definite form(s) of neurasthenia, liver disorders, kidney disorders, stomach and intestinal troubles, female disorders, melancholia, hysteria, chorea, anemia, chlorosis, sexual disorders, and so forth.

The symptoms or conditions that arise from a subnormal temperature are not necessarily in proportion to the degree of subnormal temperature. A person showing a fractional part of one degree of subnormal temperature may present problems or conditions of disease as severe as a person whose temperature is several degrees below normal.

A sufficiency of an active form of oxygen for the blood means better blood, better circulation, better assimilation, better equilibrium of body temperature, better vasomotor activity, better digestion, better elimination of waste products, less chance of auto-intoxication or toxemia (which is the keynote of many diseases), better chance for body building natural substances, and less chance of infection and disease.

After careful analytical investigation of disease, it has been demonstrated:

First: That one of the most common and important conditions that the person is called upon to correct is the weakness and incapacity produced by an impoverished or diminished blood supply.

Second: That under-oxidation produces bad health primarily because of an insufficient supply of oxygen, guaranteeing the formation of carbon monoxide, which is at once a de-oxidizer, hemo-globin destroyer, and irritant poison devitalizing the blood and paving the way to a multiplicity of acute troubles, many of which become chronic.

It has long been recognized that the atmosphere possesses the properties of blood-building, oxidation, and antisepsis. Ozone differs from atmospheric action only in degree of activity and potency. Ozone's activity makes it the greatest blood building, oxidizing, and antiseptic agent within the reach of mankind.

It has been suggested that a subnormal temperature may be a normal condition with some people. This deduction can be disproven by placing anyone with a subnormal temperature under the active influence of Ozone and having the temperature rise back to normal.

Almost all forms of nervous, functional, respiratory, and blood disorders can be successfully corrected by oxidation restoration. The effects are perfectly natural, the nerves being left calm and toned with a feeling of buoyancy and exhilaration. Oxygen restoration stimulates the vasomotor system through the nerve centers, demonstrated by increased redness of the skin, a feeling of warmth throughout the whole body, and freer elimination of waste products. The Ozone treatment shows that poor oxidation is the cause of many disorders, by reason of the fact that when the temperature is brought up to normal, problems disappear.

Oxidation is the source of life!!!

— International Oxidation Institute, ASMM

PRODUCT DESCRIPTIONS

OXY-OXC

$$\Longrightarrow \!-\!\Longleftarrow$$

*T*HE NEXT GENERATION IN SUPEROXYGENATION

Most people's primary nutritional focus is on the food and liquids they orally ingest. We take for granted that the nutrient given the highest priority by the body is oxygen, the lack of which will kill a human in a matter of minutes. Our planetary oxygen supply is becoming increasingly more toxic and its supply decreased by man-made pollutants. It is obvious that the oxygen we inhale has been greatly contaminated, especially in the inner cities. Therefore, it makes sense that enhancing one's cellular storehouse of oxygen can offset these ever-worsening conditions.

In his 1966 speech, "The Prime Cause and Prevention of Cancer," presented at the annual meeting of Nobelists in Lindau, Germany, Dr. Otto Warburg states:

Cancer, above all other diseases, has countless secondary causes. Almost anything can cause cancer but, even for cancer, there is only one prime cause. Summarized in a few words, the prime cause of cancer is the replacement of the respiration of oxygen in normal cells by a fermentation of sugar. All normal cells meet their energy needs by respiration of oxygen, whereas cancer cells meet their energy needs in great part by fermentation. All normal cells are thus obligate aerobes, whereas all cancer cells are partial anaerobes. From the standpoint of the physics and chemistry of life, this difference between normal and cancer cells is so great that one can scarcely picture a greater difference. Oxygen gas, the donor of energy in plants and animals, is dethroned in the cancer cells and replaced by an energy-yielding reaction of the lowest living forms.

A cell cannot become cancerous if its respiration is intact. Three ways are known to maintain a cell's respiration:

1) Add active groups of respiratory enzymes to your foods;

2) Saturate all growing body cells with oxygen; and

3) Keep away from external carcinogens.

Everyone knows we cannot live long without oxygen. However, many of us may be victims of a "low oxygen" condition caused by poor food, lack of exercise, polluted air, and shallow breathing. If our metabolism is not allowed to process food at the highest level of energy (high oxygen environment), our cells begin to accumulate waste products faster than the body can remove them, which in turn attracts harmful viruses and microbes (such as in flu, colds, toxic colon conditions, arterial plaque, cancer, and AIDS). If, however, the oxygen level around these anaerobic life forms is increased, they die! This may sound too simple, but there have been over 5,000 articles available in medical journals in the past 20 years regarding the action of oxygen products on pathogens.

Now you will be able to experience and benefit from Nature's simple yet powerful "product"—oxygen.

Oxy-Oxc (pronounced "OX-ee-OX-ee") is an evolutionary breakthrough in oxygen nutrition. Through an advanced proprietary process, triatomic oxygen (Ozone) is bonded through a crystal lattice matrix with magnesium peroxide, allowing a multifaceted approach to cellular oxygenation.

What are the contents of Oxy-Oxc?

A specially formulated Magnesium Peroxide Compound with Ozone/Oxygen enhancement and Vitamin C with a Bioflavonoid Complex.

What does Oxy-Oxc do?

It is a body oxygenator and energizer which detoxifies and

cleanses wastes, pathogens, and plaque from the gastro-intestinal tract, colon, arteries, blood, etc.

Why is Oxy-Oxc needed?

As a result of poor diet, lack of exercise, polluted air, shallow breathing, and stress, many of us are in a low oxygen/toxic state. This creates inefficient metabolism, causing the body to accumu late waste products faster than it can eliminate them. This then leads to a favorable environment for the proliferation of pathogenic microbes (viruses, bacteria, fungi, etc.) which, in turn, create disease conditions (flu, herpes, candida, chronic fatigue, cancer, AIDS, etc.) If, however, the oxygen level around these anaerobic pathogens is increased, they die, unable to survive the high-oxygen environment.

How does Oxy-Oxc work?

As Oxy-Oxc reaches the stomach's acid environment and continues into the bloodstream, the Vitamin C (ascorbic acid) and bioflavonoid complex break the magnesium peroxide bond, releasing the Ozone and peroxides, softening the intestinal and arterial plaque, and killing pathogenic microbes throughout the body. The Ozone and peroxides further break down into oxygen which continues to purify and energize all cells in the body. As the liquefied plaques and dead pathogens move toward leaving the body, the magnesium creates a colon flushing reaction, increasing bowel activity and preventing reabsorption of the toxins.

How is Oxy-Oxc made?

Through an advanced proprietary process, Ozone, peroxides, and magnesium are merged and bonded into a crystal lattice matrix (similar to air bubbles in ice). Vitamin C and a whole-fruit bioflavonoid complex are added to help break the bond and provide a more sustained release, thus creating optimal assimilation.

Pau D'Arco Tea &
Colon 8
Intestinal Cleanser

⇒——⋲

*P*au D'Arco tea is made from tree bark imported from South America, where it has been in use for centuries. It has only recently received recognition in this country as a powerful healing tea and safe, natural antibiotic. It is very effective in reducing congestion throughout the lymph system as well as the lungs. It also helps clear mucous and acid buildup in the body. Pau D'Arco tea is a powerful aid for the immune system and the elimination of candida overgrowth.

Instructions: Add one heaping tablespoon of Pau D'Arco tea bark to one quart of water. Bring to a boil, then simmer for 20 minutes. Strain off the bark, allow the tea to cool, and refrigerate. Drink no more than eight ounces daily, hot or cold. Continue to drink this tea after completing the candida reduction program; make it a regular part of your diet.

Colon 8 Intestinal Cleanser

Colon 8 Intestinal Cleanser is a mixture of herbs that scrubs and cleanses both the small intestine and the colon (large intestine). It will remove buildup of undigested food and mucous that may be lining the digestive and elimination system. Colon 8 is all natural and contains psyllium in a base of bentonite, oat bran, *Lactobacillus acidophilus*, whey, alfalfa, rhubarb, buckthorn, golden seal, gentian, cascara sagrada, aloe socotrina, calcium, magnesium, and other minerals natural to the herbs. This product contains no preservatives, salt, or artificial colors.

DDS ACIDOPHILUS CULTURE

$\mathcal{D}$ DS Acidophilus culture is one of just a few brands of acidophilus that is acid resistant and can survive the long journey through the digestive tract to the colon. DDS delivers one billion friendly bacteria in each capsule. These bacteria will colonize and re-establish the much needed friendly flora that may be absent due to past antibiotic use. DDS helps improve bowel movements and has an excellent cleansing effect on the liver. Acidophilus is also known to reduce blood cholesterol levels.

DDS should be taken with water only, first thing in the morning. DDS should not be taken with food or other liquids because these substances stimulate the natural stomach acids, weakening the ability of DDS to recolonize in the colon.

NOT ALL LACTOBACILLI ARE THE SAME

Although the claims and labels may look the same for Lactobacillus products, the fact is they are not the same. As a result of my studies, I've decided to use DDS Acidophilus because of its stability, potency effectiveness, and lower cost.

THERAPEUTIC EFFECTS OF DDS

Studies conducted by scientists at the University of Nebraska and Michigan State University have shown that DDS Acidophilus provides several therapeutic effects. Its specific actions include the ability to make a natural antibiotic, acidiophilin, and form lactic acid and hydrogen peroxide.

Acidiophilin, the antibiotic, is active against a wide variety of gram-positive and gram-negative bacteria, such as Streptococcus faecalis, Staphylococcus aureus, and Escherichea coli, plus a host of others.

Acidophilin has also been found to retard the growth of *Candida albicans* in the laboratory. It should be noted that yogurt has long been used as a folk remedy for vaginitis. Lactobacillus organisms are normal constituents of vaginal flora. They contribute to the maintenance of the acid pH by fermenting glycogen in the mucous to lactic acid.

Nutritional Effects

In addition to the specific therapeutic effects of DDS, Lactobacilli in general help produce B vitamins (folic acid, niacin, riboflavin, B12, B6, and pantothenic acid); aid in predigestion of proteins and formation of free amino acids; help predigest lactose (which assists people with lactose intolerance due to lack of intestinal lactase and beta-galactosidase enzymes); and have anticholesteremic and antilipedemic effects.

CAPRYSTATIN, KAPRYCIDIN-A & ORITHRUSH-D

⇁ — ⇽

*C*aprystatin contains reagent-grade caprylic acid (100 mg.) adsorbed to a non-resinous anion-exchange moiety to provide prolonged release throughout the surface area of the lower bowel. Caprystatin contains no phenols, formaldehyde, resins, or other commonly reactive ingredients. It is an effective agent to help reduce candida overgrowth in the colon.

KAPRYCIDIN-A

Kaprycidin-A contains an encapsulated form of caprylic acid (325 mg.) as calcium, magnesium, and zinc caprylates. This time-delayed caprylate complex is designed for smooth release through the gastrointestinal tract. It may be used together with Caprystatin to reduce candida overgrowth throughout the intestinal tract. Kaprycidin-A's primary action is in the small intestine.

ORITHRUSH-D

This formula includes a specially buffered solution of sorbic acid. When diluted one part Orithrush-D to 20 parts water, it is a pleasant gargle and mouth rinse. It is an effective agent for clearing candida overgrowth from the mouth, throat, and stomach. Used at full strength, it is excellent for combating vaginal yeast infection.

47

LATERO FLORA
(Bacillus laterosporus—B.O.D. Strain)

~~⟫——⟪~~

*I*n 1981, a Southern California agriculturist visiting a remote part of Iceland discovered a native who had grown the most enormous, vibrantly colored, rich tasting vegetables he had ever seen. Inquiry revealed that the soil was like no other the agriculturist knew of! Untouched by pesticides, oxides of sulphur, carbon monoxide and related gasses, airborne chemicals, and all the other common pollutants which have ravaged most of the "civilized" world's soil, this small area contained remarkably pristine, pure soil. And vegetables grown in this soil appeared to impart remarkable health benefits to those who ate them regularly.

Excited to learn more, the agriculturist returned to the U.S.A. with enough of this unique soil to study it in depth. After a series of tests, the true secret of the soil's powers of growth and regeneration was revealed: the discovery of a unique strain of bacteria, Bacillus laterosporus.

The presence of large quantities of this microorganism in the soil apparently enhanced and bolstered plant growth. It was also theorized that individuals who ate these vegetables were not only receiving beneficial nutrients, but probably were consuming significant quantities of B. laterosporus itself.

Boyd O'Donnell, now president of Bio-Genesis Corp., was intrigued by the amazing properties of B. laterosporus and continued with several years of studies and development of the special strain. He then patented it as Bacillus laterosporus B.O.D., and named the product Latero Flora. The perfected methods for growth, stabilization, and preservation of the organism have been tested through human studies in which thousands of individuals have taken the product with beneficial results.

Latero Flora is extremely effective for individuals with gastro-intestinal disturbances, food allergies, and candidiasis hypersensitivity syndrome. Latero Flora normalizes the flora in the human digestive tract, aids in digestion and toxin elimination, and discourages the growth of yeast, fungi, and other pathogenic microorganisms.

As health professionals began to use Latero Flora, thousands of patients described dramatic feelings of improvement (confirmed by lab tests), and health organizations such as the Candida Research and Information Foundation gave glowing reports from trials. No other product in existence is as effective as Latero Flora in restoring the original, desirable, bacterial balance to human intestines, thus aiding in resolving many immuno-suppressed conditions.

Since early 1989 when Latero Flora was introduced commercially, continuously growing numbers of individuals, doctors, clinics and health care professionals have praised this product.

In separate testing, Dr. Luc DeSchepper, M.D., Ph.D., C.A., studied the "before and after" symptoms of 1,500 patients. These patients suffered from chronic fatigue, along with a wide variety of immunosuppressive symptoms. Dr. DeSchepper made his report in the Townsend Letter for Doctors:

> Latero Flora has shown significant effectiveness in improving and in many cases eliminating gastrointestinal symptoms and food sensitivities, while enhancing the patient's digestive capacities... I am convinced that Latero Flora will play a very important role in fighting the scourge of this century—the suppression of our immune system.

Travacid X (HCl)

Reprinted by permission from The Spotlight, *March 23, 1987*
by Tom Valentine

🙢 — 🙠

*A*bout 50 years ago, two physicians, supported by an abundance of original research, tried to tell the medical community that hydrochloric acid (HCl), the main constituent of stomach acid, held many keys to better health.

Both Dr. Burr Ferguson and William Bryant Guy were ignored by a medical Establishment dominated by a pharmaceutical industry bent on monopolizing all medical practice and its attendant promotion of "curative" substances.

Dr. Guy wrote exhaustively of using HCl as a therapy for many deadly diseases, especially about his clinical use of injections of dilute HCl into patients' veins.

Dr. Ferguson, credited with being the first M.D. to inject dilute HCl into the veins, showed that medical science went awry when it accepted the notions of Ehrlich (antibodies and side chains). Medical science erred again when it rejected much of the work of Elie Metchnikoff, who first propounded the theory of phagocytosis to explain natural immunity.

Metchnikoff named the white blood cells "phagocytes" because they are devourers of harmful, single-celled microbes.

June Perbohner, a devoted individual researcher, has studied the literature on HCl for more than a decade and provided the *Spotlight* this detailed exclusive.

"In 1936, Dr. Ferguson wrote 'Facts and Phagocytes,' in which he outlined the work of Metchnikoff and how it affected his researches into the HCl therapy," Perbohner said. "Metchnikoff earned half the Nobel Prize for [physiology and] medicine in 1908 for his work on phagocytes as presented in his book *Immunity in Infective Diseases*. Metchnikoff also advocated [the view] that most human ailments, and even 'old age' [senescence] were due to toxicities from intestinal putrefaction."

However, Metchnikoff and his followers, who included Louis Pasteur, could not explain why the phagocytes of one sick person function so well, while another person with the same disease succumbs.

"According to Dr. Ferguson," Perbohner noted, "bacteriolysis depends upon the acid balance of the cell, the electrical potential and [other factors]. Metchnikoff said that the white cells are acid in reaction, but he had never been able to identify what acid was responsible."

However, the medical Establishment had already latched onto the theory put forth by Ehrlich and "some 200 vaccines were made by laboratories of colleges and chemical houses in the application of this hypothetical system."

Ehrlich had astounding results in the treatment of syphilis, temporarily. His arsenic compounds worked until the germs became accustomed to the poison and mercury had to be added, then bismuth. The early signs that germs would adapt and build immunity to poisons didn't deter the drug industry from making more and more poisons.

A BETTER STIMULANT

Figuring that Ehrlich had simply stimulated the phagocytes of Metchnikoff with his compounds, Ferguson sought a better chemical stimulant for the disease killing cells. He found it in nature's digestive acid.

The work of Ferguson and Guy established conclusively that

simple hydrochloric acid, HCl, served to control the vital pH factors of the body systems. Ferguson also discovered that dilute HCl injected into the blood caused an increase in the oxygen supply of the blood.

However, medical science had moved away from Metchnikoff. Administering HCl intravenously required consummate skill, so Ferguson's HCl therapy vanished.

Perbohner has been instrumental in the creation of time-release HCl "caplets," which may be taken orally and may accomplish many of the purposes of the injectable HCl. Health food stores have long offered digestive HCl pills, even though the mainstream market prefers to sell antacids to curb stomach acid, which is erroneously believed to be part of the cause of ulcers.

Infectious diseases can get their start whenever there is a shortage of HCl in the system. Germs can survive heat and cold, but seldom can they survive strong acid. Ferguson provided 25 years of clinical researches to prove his HCl thesis.

Microbial infections, such as salmonellosis (food poisoning), are common and even epidemic among Americans today because of the diminished content of HCl in the gastric juices. A recent story in *Discover* magazine related how severe the problem of salmonella poisoning has become in the United States. Resistant strains of salmonella are proliferating in poultry and meats prepared in private homes, even more so than in public eateries.

The need for a strong stomach acid is quite apparent.

HEALTHY LYMPH

Guy stressed the importance of the lymphatic system and how HCl was nature's way of keeping the lymph stream healthy and balanced. He presented his views on "the blockage of lymph channels due to changes in the hydrogenion content," and after five years of research showed that "most disease conditions, acute infections, anemias, metabolic disturbances, [etc.], are the direct result" of the changes in the pH of the lymphatic fluid. (PH is a measure of acidity.)

Guy pointed out how lymph "stasis" or blockage could seriously reduce the supply of oxygen to cells. He discovered that a subtle, but dangerous, form of lymph blockage occurred because of "mineral imbalance [and] pathological salts as seen in arthritis and gout."

Concern for the balance of minerals in the system has long been a hallmark of the so-called health faddists, while establishment medicine has downplayed the importance of such subtle balances of nature until recently.

"If oxygenation is reduced," Guy wrote, "the normal life in that group of cells slows down or ceases and abnormal metabolism begins."

Like many other great physicians of the 1920s and '30s, Guy knew that lack of oxygen for cell oxidation was the major cause of disease and aging.

Perbohner pointed out that "traveler's diarrhea" is one of the major health problems of the world and that it continues to pose puzzling problems for medical science.

"Numerous well-established facts on the relationship of reduced gastric acidity to intestinal bacterial and parasitic infection have been published," she told the *Spotlight*, "but evidence of the overall practical importance of gastric acid as it relates to immunity and intestinal bacterial and parasitic infections [is] incomplete."

She cited Dr. G.C. Cook, of the Department of Clinical and Tropical Medicine at the London School of Hygiene and Tropical Medicine, who commented as recently as 1985:

"It seems clear that far more attention was paid to gastric acid in the context of important defense mechanisms some three or four decades ago than is the case today. Altered emphasis has resulted from the explosion of interest in the immunological defense mechanisms which protect the gastrointestinal tract."

Cook also wrote: "Although the study of host defenses against intestinal infections is now dominated by immunologists, there is an important place for further research on gastric acidity in the context of infection."

Perbohner added: "It is timely to suggest that clinical research be undertaken on hydrogen and chloride ions in the context of so-called traveler's diarrhea and other related conditions."

Testimonials already abound to the efficacy of time-released HCl and sodium-chloride oxygen compounds in the prevention of food poisoning and traveler's diarrhea. Both are ideas from the 1930s coming back.

It is interesting that a call can be made these days for more research into gastric acid. Why was so much quality research ignored 50 years ago?

COENZYME Q10

⋙ —— ⋘

Coenzyme Q10 (CoQ for short) is an important vitamin-like nutrient that functions biochemically as an anti-oxidant and free radical scavenger. But CoQ has a specific biochemical role of major importance. CoQ is essential for the production of cellular energy, and its role in producing energy in heart cells is of special interest. The steady stream of energy that is required to sustain life absolutely depends on each cell having adequate levels of CoQ.

This nutrient has become the focus of intense worldwide study. Hundreds of papers extolling the benefits of CoQ have been published in Japan, Europe, the former Soviet Union, and more recently in the U.S. CoQ is available from foods such as beef, spinach, and sardines. However, the body's ability to synthesize CoQ from foods diminishes with age and, furthermore, foods lose CoQ with processing and storage. CoQ is used throughout the world as a supplement to treat or prevent heart disease and high blood pressure, enhance the immune system, and slow the aging process. In Japan alone, more than 12 million people take daily doses of CoQ prescribed by their physicians for prevention and treatment of heart and circulatory disorders.

Animal studies conducted by Dr. Emile Bliznakov, Scientific Director of the Lupus Research Institute, have shown that mean life span can be increased significantly with CoQ. His experiments were conducted with mice whose ages were comparable to humans in their late sixties or early seventies. Within three to four months, the CoQ-supplemented mice were noticeable for their greater vigor and mobility, more lustrous hair, brighter eyes, and the absence of the normal signs of advanced age which were readily apparent in the control group. The life span of the CoQ-supplemented mice was twice as long as their predicted life expectancy.

The dual role of CoQ as an energy carrier and antioxidant may help account for its potential benefit for virtually every category of cell, tissue, and organ function. CoQ is a safe nutrient that is without significant side effects. CoQ has passed the toxicity studies required by the FDA for clinical trials in the United States. Topics of current research interest in CoQ include lupus, AIDS, diabetes, periodontal disease, *Candida albicans* infection, Parkinson's disease, and muscular dystrophy.

BENEFITS
Coenzyme Q10:
- Has proven of benefit in a variety of cardiovascular disorders.
- Enhances survival of heart tissue under low oxygen conditions and excessive loads.
- Has been shown in studies to have a stabilizing effect on heart rhythms.
- Can be effective in normalizing blood pressure in hypertensive individuals.
- May significantly enhance athletic performance.
- Helps improve oxygen transport and consumption and increase workload capacity.
- Has been shown to increase resistance to viral infections.
- Helps protect against chemically caused cancers.
- May dramatically increase antibody levels and stimulate the immune system.
- Has been proven effective in the treatment of obesity.
- Offers protection against inflammatory gum diseases.
- Has proven useful against diabetes and certain hearing disorders.
- Has been found effective in double-blind clinical studies in the treatment of AIDS.

IMMUNO-QUEST

$$\Rightarrow\!\!-\!\!\Leftarrow$$

*I*t has long been recognized that the healthy body's defense mechanisms consist of white blood cells, lymph cells, and antibodies. White blood cells are found throughout the blood, serving to destroy bacteria, while lymph cells destroy viruses and antibodies, protecting us from foreign proteins and matter that are associated with bacteria.

Viruses and bacteria are opportunistic living organisms that prey upon us when our immune system is weak. Factors that can affect our immunity are poor diet, stress, lack of exercise, tobacco and alcohol use, and even some medications. The temperature, pH, and low energy level of our body when we are in a run-down state creates the perfect environment for viruses and bacteria to flourish. When they proliferate sufficiently, our body's immune defenses break down and we develop the physical symptoms of illness. Such illnesses include the common cold and flu, and the range of infections from herpes to AIDS.

Drugs relieve only the physical symptoms of infection, often times making the situation worse by killing the bacteria and leaving their dead bodies in our tissues to serve as breeding material for new bacteria and viruses. This creates a vicious cycle of illness until our immune defense system becomes damaged and chronic disease sets in. Such diseases include allergies, lupus, arthritis, chronic infections, and cancer.

Scientists are daily gaining a better understanding of the immune system and what it takes to biochemically aid and support

59

its function. Many of these biochemical components are being found in vitamins, minerals and herbs, nutrients that are essential in nourishing our bodies.

Immuno-Quest combines essential nutrients to reinforce and stimulate our bodily defenses. These are as follows:

Vitamin C: This essential vitamin is always depleted in the tissues during illness. It stimulates the production of antibodies and white blood cells, and is deadly to all viruses. It is also important to the body's recuperative powers and vascular strength.

Vitamin A: Vitamin A is also essential to the production of antibodies, white blood cells and lymphocytes. As with Vitamin C, the level of Vitamin A drops sharply during infections. Vitamin A also promotes the repair of tissues damaged by illness and stress.

Zinc: Experiments performed by DuPont scientists showed that by adding zinc to tissue cultures the formation of bacteria and viruses was immediately inhibited. Zinc has been widely used commercially in antibacterial preparations because of its bacterial inhibiting properties. Zinc is one of our most important minerals, having over 32 functions in our bodies.

Pantothenic Acid (Vitamin B5): This nutrient is necessary for the production of cortisone, an anti-inflammatory agent in the body. Vitamins B5 and B6 also help to promote production of antibodies and white blood cells.

Vitamin B12 and *RNA*: These two nutrients support the body as antitoxins during chronic infections such as mononucleosis and hepatitis. Their effect is enhanced by Vitamins C and A, bioflavonoids, and other nutrients.

Coenzyme Q10: This nutrient is found in all tissues and has many functions, primarily antioxidant in nature. Studies have shown that it retards cellular destruction from aging and stress, thus enhancing healing. Other studies have shown that supplemental Coenzyme Q10 increases immunoglobulin and the germ-killing ability of white blood cells.

L-Lysine: An essential amino acid, l-lysine is principally an antiviral agent. It has been used successfully in the treatment of herpes and herpeto-viruses such as chicken pox. Combined with Coenzyme Q10 and Vitamin C, l-lysine has a synergistic effect.

Glandular Extracts: Commonly known as protomorphigens, freeze-dried glandulars have been widely used. In medicine, thyroid extract is used quite frequently. In nutrition, glandulars add micronutrients that support the activity of their targeted gland. The immune glands are the thymus, spleen, lymph, and lung.

Herbal Concentrates: Echinacea is one of the most outstanding herbs for the immune system, activating white blood and lymph cells. It is an effective antibacterial and antiviral agent possessing similar activity to interferon. It is also a good blood purifier, toning those organs that filter impurities from the blood. Alfalfa, chlorophyll, and kelp are powerful herbs that act to normalize the pH balance, creating a nutritional environment for proper vitamin and mineral absorption. These herbs also help to "sweeten" the digestive tract, removing and neutralizing toxic mucous.

NATUR-EARTH

⋙——⋘

*A*N AMAZING NEW BREAKTHROUGH IN IMMUNE
STIMULATION AND HEALING

Scientists are working on "grooming" various non-native
microorganisms to perform specific tasks in the human body, such
as destroying certain viruses, or stimulating specific functions
within the immune system. In several instances, great strides have
been made in these areas—one of which has been in the development and use of *soil-based microorganisms* for promoting overall
healing in human beings, as well as for stimulating powerful
responses unlike anything ever reported.

Later you will learn the inside details on a unique new immune-
therapeutic product called Natur-Earth, which utilizes soil-based
microorganisms in its makeup. But first, here's a brief explanation
of what soil-based microorganisms are, and what they do.

SBOS IN THE HUMAN DIET

Most Americans don't realize it, but many forms of SBOs, as
well as their enzyme, hormone, and nutrient byproducts, are
unknowingly ingested into the human system—with very beneficial effects—when fresh raw fruits and vegetables are eaten. This
was especially true in the 19th century, when America was basically
one large rural farming community and the ingestion of fresh raw
fruits and vegetables—often straight from the fields or directly
from family gardens—was commonplace.

Today, however, human ingestion of SBOs and their beneficial byproducts is far less common. This is because modern agricultural techniques (including the over-application of powerful pesticides, fungicides, and germicidal agents) and heat-based food processing techniques tend to kill off SBOs on fruits and vegetables, as well as destroy the beneficial enzyme, hormone, and nutrient by-products normally released by SBOs and absorbed by the food plants as part of the normal growth cycle. Nonetheless, SBOs and their beneficial byproducts still manage to find their way into the human system today in this country, though with far less frequency than in times past.

It is because of this that a number of nutritionists working on the cutting edge of orthomolecular medicine now speculate that the declining digestive intake of SBOs and their enzyme, hormone, and nutrient by-products is one of the chief reasons Americans tend to experience far more bowel and digestive systems problems than do the people of other countries, where modern high-tech farming and food processing techniques have yet to replace family farms and gardens. In other countries, SBO intake is markedly higher via the intake of fresh raw plant life, and digestive tract problems are correspondingly lower!

The Making of Natur-Earth

In the late 1980s a reclusive scientist by the name of Peter Smith was on a trip overseas. While hiking through a pristine area of a foreign country [which, to this day, he won't name—Ed.], he spotted some large clumps on the ground, which he recognized as huge colonies of soil-based microorganisms. Smith was intrigued by the unusual nature of what he saw, and brought some of the microorganisms back into the United States for research and experimentation. Later, he returned several times to the original location to obtain additional samples.

For the next few years, Smith conducted phased studies of the soil-based microorganisms he had discovered. Phase #1 was to identify the various strains of SBOs found living in the clumps.

Phase #2 was to determine if the SBOs were toxic or pathogenic. Phase #3 was to ascertain what, if any, beneficial value these soil-based bacteria might be able to impart to living things, particularly animals and humans.

After considerable painstaking and detailed research, the specific strains of soil-based bacilli Smith had discovered were identified. Toxicity tests proved negative on fingerling fish. In fact, far from being harmed, the fish began rapidly increasing in size when taking the bacteria. Toxicity tests were then carefully conducted on rodents and other members of the animal kingdom with equally positive results. There was nothing in the bacteria toxic to animals. At the same time, extensive botany tests were conducted which showed that the bacteria were amazingly beneficial to plants and soil.

Smith became the first human being to use the bacterial culture himself—first using it topically on open wounds, and later ingesting it. Again there were no toxic reactions to the bacteria, and there were no harmful side effects. In fact, it seemed to give increasingly positive health results as more and more of the organisms were consumed.

According to the source material we were able to obtain for this report, Smith's research was conducted in the laboratories of several major California universities. He collaborated with top professors and other research experts, and was able to utilize the facilities of the laboratories freely, as well as the computer data banks.

In the course of his research and experimentation, Smith and his laboratory coworkers were able to perfect a process for selectively breeding superior strains of the tiny microorganism, as well as for "grooming" them until they had a culture that, when ingested by humans, produced very specific and quite startling healing and immune-stimulating results, with absolutely no toxic effects or other unwanted side effects. The combined corporate effort of Smith and his university colleagues ultimately resulted in the development of the amazing Natur-Earth food supplement product.

Natur-Earth is manufactured as a gray-black powder. The powder, which is composed chiefly of a broad array of specific micronutrients and phytoplankton, acts as a *substrate* for live soil-based microorganisms. Through a special process, the SBOs are kept in a dormant state within the powder, and do not become active until introduced into a aqueous solution such as water or juice. Because of this, Natur-Earth boasts a shelf-life of over five years at room temperature, and even longer if refrigerated.

SECRET PROCESS

In the course of our research on this product, we discovered that Smith holds no patent to Natur-Earth, nor to the various processes he developed in order to selectively breed and "groom" the soil-based microorganisms. Nor has he patented his technique for putting the organisms into the dormant state which gives them such an unusually long shelf life. According to our sources, this is because he wants to prevent his product from being duplicated or stolen.

To this day, Smith will not identify the original soil-based organisms he discovered, nor discuss his processes for selectively breeding and grooming the superior strains from the original cultures.

DRAMATIC HEALING RESULTS!

Nonetheless, in spite of all the secrecy surrounding Natur-Earth, the product has enjoyed over 12 years of continuous—albeit very quiet—use by the relatively small number of people who have been fortunate enough to hear about it. In that time, no toxic side effects have ever been reported. What *has* been reported over the course of the past 12 years are dramatic cases of remission from some of the most serious illnesses and chronic degenerative diseases known to man, including candida.

What's more, users of Natur-Earth report numerous other ongoing health benefits, such as virtual immunity from colds and flu, stronger digestive capabilities, elimination of constipation and other chronic digestive disorders, increased and/or stabilized metabolism, increased energy levels, increased physical strength, greater resistance to inflammation, quicker resistance to infection, quicker healing of wounds, increased mental clarity, and much, much more.

We were able to examine the results of specific tests, as well as scientific laboratory analysis performed on the product, which revealed the specific actions through which Natur-Earth is able to stabilize the metabolism in human beings, radically boost nutritional assimilation, and simultaneously amplify the human immune system to such a degree that illness and disease can be warded off indefinitely, and even reversed if already in progress.

This information gives a startling insight into what makes Natur-Earth such a remarkable therapeutic product. We'll give you some of the specific details in just a moment, but first, here's a basic outline of how Natur-Earth works when taken orally, as well as a brief description of the five main functions of the SBOs contained in Natur-Earth.

How It Works: A Basic Outline

When Natur-Earth is ingested, it moves from the stomach to the intestinal tract and forms colonies of beneficial SBOs along the way, which attach themselves to the intestinal wall. Then, as food works its way through the gastrointestinal system, it drags some of the bacteria from these colonies further "down the line," these bacteria also attaching to the intestinal wall. Within a short period of time, the microorganism attachment to the intestinal wall encompasses literally the entire length of the gastrointestinal tract.

The SBOs in Natur-Earth grow and multiply into large colonies wherever they attach to the intestinal wall. Once established, they quickly begin producing an environment which dramatically stimulates the body's ability to absorb and utilize crucial nutrients, while simultaneously ridding the intestinal tract of both putrefaction and pathogenic (i.e., disease-causing) organisms.

Here are five of the main functions conducted by the SBOs once they are integrated into the human intestinal system through ingestion as a food supplement.

Function #1: Once the SBOs have established their colonies in the digestive tract, they immediately begin eliminating all accumulated putrefaction in which harmful pathogenic organisms thrive. The SBOs have the ability to get in behind putrefaction that has stuck to the walls of the colon and other areas of the intestinal tract and devour it. Excess putrefaction is dislodged by the SBOs and then flushed out of the intestinal tract by the normal eliminative process.

Function #2: The SBOs also go to work breaking down hydrocarbons. With this unique ability, all foods are broken down into their most basic elements, allowing almost total absorption through the digestive system, thereby dramatically increasing overall nutrition and rapidly enhancing cellular growth and development. This process also vastly aids the digestive system in the process of elimination because of the unusually thorough and complete manner in which foods are broken down by the SBOs. As a major side benefit, constipation is eliminated almost overnight.

Function #3: While in the digestive tract, the SBOs produce specific proteins which act as antigens. These in turn stimulate the immune system to produce huge quantities of antibodies over and above that which the immune system would normally have available for use. This vastly increased antibody output dramatically amplifies the immune system's ability to ward off disease and illness. Plus, it enhances the immune system's ability to battle virtually any disease or illness already afflicting the body. Because of this factor, which we'll explain in-depth, many individuals using Natur-Earth have reported amazing healing results from diseases.

Function #4: The SBOs are extremely aggressive against pathological molds, yeast, fungi, and viruses. They quickly engulf and ingest harmful microbes such as *Candida Albicans, Candida Parasylois, Penicillin Frequency, Penicillin Natatum, Muco Rasmosue,*

Aspergillus Niger, and many others, which would otherwise infect the body and cause serious illness and even chronic degenerative disease. In eliminating pathogenic microbes, the SBOs end up allowing the overworked immune system to rest and gain strength.

Function #5: The SBOs work in a symbiotic relation to somatic cells. They metabolize proteins for the cells and simultaneously help rid them of toxic wastes, thereby dramatically boosting normal cellular functions which are the very basis of all human health.

Chiefly because of these five specific functions of the SBOs contained in Natur-Earth, dramatic healing and immune-stimulation are being achieved for people around the world who are quietly using this unique and exclusive new therapeutic food supplement. But the truly fascinating immune-stimulating effects of the SBOs can only be fully realized when one looks at the data produced by ongoing laboratory tests being conducted by some of the world's top scientists and immune system experts.

NATUR-EARTH AND THE HUMAN IMMUNE SYSTEM: THE INSIDE DETAILS

"When I first heard about this product, well frankly, I thought to myself 'this is probably just snake oil.' I was very suspicious. Then I heard how people with arthritis were being helped, and people with Lou Gehrig's disease. And people with various kinds of cancer. So I went out to Los Angeles and interviewed people who had used it, and looked at their medical histories, and I became a believer... Without a doubt, people are being helped."

—Dr. Don Boys, PhD

"I didn't believe what I was reading about this product. I started studying it. Soon, I could see the logic behind how and why it works. The first patient we put on this product was a man with a serious bladder and kidney infection, who also had enlargement of the prostate and was scheduled for prostate surgery. Within four days of taking the product there was no more infection, so the surgery was temporarily postponed. Two weeks later the patient was re-examined and there was no more enlargement of the prostrate. The surgery was cancelled... This is just one example of the amazing results we've witnessed with this product. We've recorded remissions from various diseases beginning within three days to four weeks after using this product... Cancers, Parkinson's disease, glaucoma, nervous disorders, high cholesterol levels, and many other conditions and diseases have responded successfully to this product."

—Dr. Phyllis Wilson Confer
Marko, Indiana

"I had breast cancer that had metastasized to the bone. By the time it was found, it was simply too late for conventional therapy. It was advanced to the point of being a death sentence. I was in a lot of pain... I started taking the product in November, and within weeks I felt decreased pain—in fact, about 95 percent less pain. Since then the central mass of cancer in my breast has decreased from a two and one-half inch mass to the size of a small pea."

—Dr. A. Johnson
(City/State withheld on request)

"I have been afflicted with arthritis for nearly 20 years, and in recent years have had to use a wheelchair to get around the house. I started taking this product twice daily in orange juice. It took about two or three weeks for the pain to go away. I find it better to take than the pills and other medication the doctors give me, as there are no side effects. The doctor's medicine gave me an ulcer. But this product is the best thing I've ever tried."

—I. C. (age 74), Texas

"My health for over one month's time was very poor. I was operating on about 25 to 50 percent of my energy level. I had swollen glands and a sore throat... The doctor's statement—'you just have to ride it out because I have nothing to give you to make you feel better.' I spoke with my neighbor, and he told me about your product. He gave me some to try, told me to take it twice a day. Within 12 hours my sore throat was gone, and 24 hours later my glands stopped hurting, and within 48 hours my energy level was back to normal! It was definitely a miracle cure for me."

—M. M., California

"For 13 years I wrestled to find a way to stabilize and hopefully heal one of my children who had uncontrollable epilepsy which traditional Western medication did not help. Last year, while visiting with a man who has been called one of the top five biochemists in the world, at his prestigious clinic in Key Biscayne, Florida, I was introduced to a product he dubbed 'black gold'... When I began giving my epileptic child this product, the petit mal seizures, which had been continuous for 13 years, stopped literally overnight... Could these beneficial microorganisms emit substances which are useful to the human intestine, and work against foreign matter or other debris found in the intestine? Could these microorganisms, as they grow in colonies, emit substances which stimulate the body's response to produce antibodies which are an immune simulator, which in turn amplify and stabilize the body's immune system? All I know for sure is that this product knocked out my child's petit mal seizures, and has increased my energy level and stamina."

—R. E. McMaster
Publisher, *The Reaper*

As we've stated earlier, the amazing immune-stimulating benefits produced by the actions of the SBOs in Natur-Earth have been demonstrated in literally hundreds of individual cases over the past 12 years. The examples above are just a small fraction of personal testimonials from users of this amazing product. Clinical trials now underway in Mexico, Venezuela, Spain, and other countries will provide even more detailed documentation of the amazing healing effects being experienced by individuals when this product is used regularly.

In the meantime, laboratory examinations have provided some fascinating in-depth insights into how it works in the human body, and why such dramatic healing and immune-stimulation benefits are being experienced by so many individuals with such a diversity of illnesses and disease.

In the course of laboratory analysis, three totally unique immune-stimulation actions have been discovered. Each of these three specific actions constitute major new breakthroughs in ortho-molecular medicine that offer profound ramifications for modern medical science. To our knowledge, medical science so far has produced nothing that can duplicate these three extremely powerful immune-stimulating actions, which are as follows:

Action #1: Stimulation of the Body's Natural Alpha Interferon Production

According to Dr. Peter Rothschild, who has conducted in-depth laboratory analysis of Natur-Earth and the beneficial SBOs, once they are firmly established in the gastrointestinal tract, they stimulate the body's own natural production of *alpha-interferon*.

Alpha-interferon is a paramount polypeptide—a protein form molecule—that was discovered in the human body in 1956 and has been proven to be a key regulator of the human immune response. Since its discovery, it has been universally acknowledged by science that the development of a widely useable man-made form of alpha-interferon would embody profound hope for the cure of many diseases in the future. Unfortunately, to date science has failed to develop a form of alpha-interferon that could live up to the high expectations held for it since its discovery in the human body.

Medical science's recombinantly-derived alpha-interferon has limited applications, with limited beneficial effects. For one, the extreme dosages (i.e., multi-million unit daily doses) required in order to stimulate immune response in humans have proven to be highly toxic. Achieving a pure form of the element has also been a major problem for medical science. What's more, the man-made alpha-interferon has proven to be prohibitively costly to manufacture and utilize, with individual treatments costing thousands upon thousands of dollars.

Additionally distressing is the fact that the recombinantly-derived interferons used by medical science today have only a single species of alpha-interferon which exerts a very low immune-stimulation response, whereas the interferons produced naturally by the human body are *multi-species* in nature. The healthy human leukocyte cell can produce up to *twenty* different sub-species of alpha-interferon and exert an *extremely aggressive* immune response.

Moreover, science now knows that the reason the human body produces so many different subspecies of alpha-interferon is because different subspecies are required to protect cells against different viruses and other antigens. No single sub-species of endogenous (i.e., body-produced) alpha-interferon can protect the human system against the variety of harmful invaders with which it must regularly contend. Therefore, the limited immune benefits of the expensive, single-species alpha-interferon produced by medical science simply cannot hold a candle to the vast immune benefits of the multi-species of alpha-interferon produced naturally by the human body itself.

In laboratory tests performed by Dr. Rothschild, the actions of the soil-based organisms contained in Natur-Earth have been shown to uniquely stimulate the human body's own production *of not less than 16 of the possible 20 subspecies of natural human alpha-*

interferon! Dr. Rothschild speculates that it is this incredible stimulation of the body's production of its own natural alpha-interferon which has caused Natur-Earth to be so highly effective in the treatment of a wide variety of chronic degenerative diseases such as chronic fatigue syndrome, viral herpes, hepatitis-B and C, influenza, and much more. To date, we know of no other product which can achieve such a profound immune-stimulating action.

What's more, according to Dr. Rothschild, "The anti-viral activity stimulated by the SBOs in Natur-Earth is even more clear, for the virus-antagonistic effect of alpha-interferon has long been documented by worldwide scientific investigation... *Our research has identified over 50 different immune modulating effects to date...* This research has produced ample evidence indicating Natur-Earth exerts a potent immune-modulatory influence with significant clinical benefits to patients who suffer from a variety of viral aggressions or other immunopathic, degenerative conditions."

Additionally, Dr. Rothschild found that, "Since Natur-Earth does not contain any toxic, addictive or otherwise dangerous substance, it is totally harmless and provides the particular elements required for stimulating both the body's T-cell production and their quality. It also eliminates the need for poisonously high-dose and inordinately expensive alpha-interferon injections."

In short, it now appears that the SBOs in Natur-Earth are unique in that their actions in the human gastrointestinal tract are somehow *able to stimulate the body's own production of the vast majority of subspecies of its own natural alpha-interferon,* thereby dramatically enhancing the immune system's ability to ward off illness and disease. T-lymphocyte production is greatly boosted and the anti-viral activity of the immune system is vastly stimulated as a direct effect of increased alpha-interferon production.

What's more, because the alpha-interferon produced as a result of the ingestion of Natur-Earth is endogenous, it is also far more assimilable by the human immune system than medical science's recombinantly-derived alpha-interferon. And the overwhelming problems of purity and toxicity are completely eliminated through the use of Natur-Earth, since it merely stimulates the body to produce its own naturally pure forms.

Lastly, instead of medical science having to indulge in vastly ineffective immune system treatments costing thousands upon thousands of dollars as they do now with their recombinantly-derived alpha-interferon, dramatic and highly effective immune-stimulating results can be achieved in the human body for a tiny fraction of the cost through the use of Natur-Earth!

Action #2: Stimulation of B-lymphocytes and Related Antibody Production

Once established in the gastrointestinal tract, the SBOs in Natur-Earth quickly begin producing a protein biomass which the body reacts to as an antigen (i.e., a foreign substance). In response to the antigenic biomass, the body immediately begins producing large quantities of *B-lymphocytes*, which in turn produce large quantities of *antibodies.*

According to Dr. Rothschild's extensive laboratory experimentation and analysis, the antibodies produced by the immune system in reaction to the antigenic biomass from the SBOs are *extremely unique* in that they are "non-addressed" antibodies. That is, they have not been "pre-programmed" by the immune system to attack any specific infection or pathogenic agent.

Instead, huge pools of antibodies are produced as long as the SBOs are ingested on a regular basis, *and they are kept in reserve by the body for use whenever needed by the immune system.* If an actual infection takes hold, or a specific pathogen invades the body, the immune system then instantly—at a moment's notice—"imprints" this large reservoir of otherwise innocuous antibodies with the precise information needed to attack the specific infection or pathogenic agent at hand. Then, quite rapidly and with incredible effectiveness, the antibodies go to work attacking the infection or pathogen at once, and wipes it out.

As explained by Dr. Rothschild, "The beauty of it all is that this huge reservoir of extra antibodies is always on hand for the immune system to utilize; as long as the individual is ingesting the SBOs regularly, the effectiveness of the human immune system is vastly enhanced. This extra contingent of antibodies is always there to attack infection, therefore the immune system does not have to work anywhere near as hard as it normally would to fight off infection."

In a nutshell, it appears that the SBOs in Natur-Earth stimulate the human immune system to produce huge pools of extra antibodies—unique, *nonspecific* antibodies which the immune system can encode whenever necessary to fight off many different types of infection or pathogenic agents. Thanks to these billions of extra antibodies, the human system can be kept far safer from infection or invading pathogens than ever before. With this unusual immuno-stimulatory effect, the human body can now act far more effectively to protect itself from infection or invading pathogens.

Action #3: Crucial Lactoferrin Supplementation to the Human Body

Dr. Rothschild has discovered that one of the most amazing aspects of the SBOs used in Natur-Earth is their ability to produce lactoferrin in the human body as a by-product of their metabolism. Lactoferrin, an iron-binding protein, is specifically utilized to retrieve iron from the foods we ingest, and then deliver the iron wherever it is needed by the body. Because the affinity of lactoferrin for iron is very high, it is able to retain and transport iron even through the harsh gastric environment, so it can be delivered to the small intestine where it is absorbed by specific receptors on the epithelial cells.

Unfortunately, lactoferrin levels are often not high enough in the human body for a variety of reasons. As a consequence, many people have trouble properly assimilating the iron they've ingested through the foods they eat. And because the body is not assimilating iron properly, symptoms of *iron deficiency* appear, even though plenty of iron is being ingested on a daily basis.

This problem is further compounded today because Americans are literally inundated with advertisements from vitamin manufacturers telling them they need to take iron supplements. What's more, many doctors tell their patients they are suffering from "iron poor blood" and need to ingest supplemental iron tablets. In reality, what most Americans need to do is increase their bodily levels of lactoferrin, so that the iron from the foods they eat—*which is more than adequate for the human system*—is more thoroughly assimilated.

In fact, as Dr. Peter Rothschild points out in his recently published research report on the *Biology of Lactoferrin*, "Of the 750 million people who suffer from iron deficiency symptoms, less than half of them suffer from any actual lack of iron in their diet." Instead, he explains, their iron deficiency symptoms are due chiefly to metabolic problems (such as those caused by insufficient levels of lactoferrin) that hinder the assimilation of iron from the food they eat, or because of the low bio-accessibility of the ingested iron.

Of course, this creates a serious problem when individuals suffering from alleged "iron deficiency" begin taking iron supplements. The additional iron being ingested does absolutely nothing to alleviate the iron deficiency symptoms because it, too, remains unassimilated by the body. As a result, the body becomes inundated with iron that it simply cannot assimilate and utilize.

Worse yet, excess iron soon begins to support the growth of infectious agents throughout the human body, due to the fact that harmful bacteria, yeasts, viruses, and other parasites have a continuous metabolic need for iron, and tend to thrive in an iron-rich environment!

On the other hand, when iron is carried through the body by lactoferrin, as it is meant to be, more than 95 percent of it is assimilable. Lactoferrin carries the iron directly to specific receptor sites in the body where it can be absorbed and utilized. Because it is attached to lactoferrin, iron cannot be absorbed and utilized by the bacteria, viruses, yeasts, and other harmful parasites that require it for their metabolism.

What all of this means, according to Dr. Rothschild, is that "One of lactoferrin's primary functions in the human body is to act as a first line of defense against all invading pathogens."

In short, lactoferrin not only makes the iron we absorb from food readily assimilable by the human body (thereby eliminating iron deficiency symptoms), it also deprives infectious organisms of this crucial element needed for their survival and growth. In a sense, it *starves to death* harmful organisms in the human body by depriving them of iron, thus short-circuiting their metabolic functions!

As mentioned earlier, Dr. Rothschild's research has shown that the SBOs in Natur-Earth produce lactoferrin in the human body as a result of their own metabolism. So by taking Natur-Earth regularly, your body will be far better able to absorb, assimilate, and utilize the iron supplied by the food you eat. Iron supplements should become completely unnecessary, once your body begins taking advantage of the increased levels of lactoferrin supplied by Natur-Earth, which reduces fatigue.

SUMMARY OF NATUR-EARTH'S UNIQUE IMMUNE-STIMULATING ACTIONS

In summary, the beneficial SBOs used in Natur-Earth provide an exclusive triple action level of immune-stimulation that is not available through any other therapeutic development we know of.

1) They stimulate the body's own natural alpha-interferon production, thereby providing markedly increased T-lymphocyte levels, dramatically increased viral resistance, and a high level of protection against chronic degenerative disease unattainable by modern medical science up until now;

2) They also stimulate the production of crucial B-lymphocytes and related antibodies, providing the immune system with a huge extra reservoir of anti-pathogenic defense organisms that are available for use at a moment's notice; and,

3) They directly produce much needed lactoferrin for the human body, which helps protect it from invading pathogens by

depriving them of the iron they need in order to survive in the human system.

MORE AMAZING THERAPEUTIC BENEFITS

In addition to all of these immuno-therapeutic benefits, the SBOs in Natur-Earth also produce and/or stimulate a vast number of other important health-related benefits. Dr. Rothschild's laboratory research on Natur-Earth has shown that it produces at least 50 distinct beneficial immune-modeling effects alone. In addition, it also directly produces and/or stimulates a number of crucial cellular health benefits.

STIMULATES CELLULAR SELF-REPAIR

For example, as a result of their action in the human system, the SBOs contained in Natur-Earth produce a wide array of DNA with their correspondent RNA. The DNA/RNA produced by the SBOs is of the specific type which is very desirable for the human body, because it carries naturally-coded instructions for the activation of self-repair in certain human cells.

It is believed that this specific factor is the reason many users of Natur-Earth have reported incredible accelerations of wound healing, particularly in regard to severe skin burns, ulcers, surgical incisions, and even wounds that had become infected. Apparently, the DNA/RNA produced by the SBOs helps aid the body in activating cellular self-repair by making available a pool of extra DNA/RNA that is immediately available to the cells, and can go right to work whenever injury occurs.

PROVIDES POWERFUL ANTI-OXIDANTS

But the therapeutic benefits don't end with the production of cell-repairing DNA and RNA. Another interesting action of the SBOs in Natur-Earth is that they produce SOD (Super Oxide Dismutase) as a by-product of their metabolism in the human system. SOD is a powerful enzyme and cellular anti-oxidant that acts as a super-scavenger of dangerous free radicals by ferreting out and destroying them throughout the body.

This is important, because free radicals are highly active and unstable and will attack any molecule in the body. Organ or tissue damage can occur whenever production of free radicals exceeds that of scavenger enzymes, such as SOD, which are the first-line defense system of the body's tissues.

But because very few foods contain SOD, our bodies are often deficient in this all-important enzyme. Thus, the damaging effects of free radicals (such as superoxide radical O_2, which induce cancer and a variety of painful inflammatory diseases as well) often goes unchecked. By introducing SOD into the human system on a regular basis, such as through the use of Natur-Earth, many dangerous free radicals can be easily extinguished before they harm the cells.

What's more, studies conducted at Johns Hopkins University have shown that SOD eliminates or greatly reduces tissue damage in the heart (particularly after a heart attack). Plus, it can also reduce tissue damage in the kidneys, the intestines, the pancreas, and the skin. This is because the enzymatic activity of SOD greatly increases the efficiency of energy production within the cells of organ tissues, allowing them to nourish and repair themselves at a more efficient and effective rate.

By using Natur-Earth on a regular basis, your body will be assured of receiving beneficial amounts of this all-important enzyme, as well as literally dozens of others.

CORRECTS NUTRIENT ABSORPTION DEFICIENCIES

In addition to all of the startling health benefits detailed above, Natur-Earth also provides a unique level of micronutrient support of the human body unparalleled in any other therapeutic product we've ever investigated. More importantly, this special level of micronutrient support acts to correct nutrient absorption deficiencies in the body, *thereby giving the human system the ability to obtain all of the nutrients it needs from daily food intake*, rather than having to depend upon a plethora of nutrient supplements. Here's how it works.

Most nutrient supplement products are based upon the premise that the human body is simply not getting enough nutrients from the food it ingests on a daily basis. Therefore, most of today's nutrient supplement products are designed to inundate the body with medium-to-large dosages of nutrients in order to make up for the alleged deficit of nutrients in the food supply.

But this form of nutrient supplementation rarely works well because the premise it is based upon is patently false. As Dr. Rothschild points out in his recent research report entitled *Bioactive Micronutrient Minerals: Biological Response Modifiers*, "A specific or multiple mineral deficit in a human body usually does NOT imply that there is a corresponding deficit of these minerals in the individual's daily nutrition... Instead, the real problem in such individuals is a chronic absorption deficiency."

In other words, as a general rule there are plenty of nutrients in the foods we eat, but due to aging, abuse or other factors, our bodies are having a difficult time *absorbing* these nutrients. So, in reality, flooding the human body with high-dose nutrient supplements is of little benefit because the whole problem in the first place is the body's inability to properly absorb nutrients!

That's where Natur-Earth is distinctly different—and far more effective—than all other nutrient supplements. Instead of inundating the body with overly-high levels of supplemental nutrients, it instead provides a wide array of key nutrients in special *micronutrient dosages*. These tiny microscopic dosages are so easy to assimilate that they act as veritable *blueprints* for the body, showing it how to properly absorb other nutrients already available in quite adequate levels through daily food intake.

In a very real sense, the special microscopic dosages of nutrients supplied in Natur-Earth act as biological "data," literally providing the cells of the human body with an "absorption pattern" which shows them how to effectively assimilate and utilize the higher levels of nutrients contained in most foods.

Dr. Rothschild's research has revealed that some of the key micronutrients made available to the body through the ingestion of Natur-Earth are actually produced as by-products of the metabolism of the SBOs once they enter the body. Other micronutrients are contained *within the SBOs themselves,* and are made available to the human body as the SBOs die off and the body digests them. And still other micronutrients are contained in the freshly-cultivated phyto-plankton (i.e., blue-green algae) cells used in Natur-Earth as a nutrient substrate.

There are at least 71 naturally occurring nutrients available in Natur-Earth, or provided as a by-product of the metabolism of the SBOs contained in the product. These include numerous beneficial pigments such as chlorophyll and phytocyanin, plus amino acids, vitamins (including the crucial B-12), minerals, key enzymes (including SOD and bromelain), nucleic acids, proteins, and more.

Additionally, Natur-Earth contains the immune-stimulating, cancer-preventing, vitamin A precursor known as beta-carotene. It also supplies the body with Gamma Linolenic Acid (GLA), which is one of the essential fatty acids without which the body could not produce hormones. In fact, without GLA the endocrine system cannot even function. [Note the human body is unable to synthesize GLA, and often has a hard time extracting it from foods. Natur-Earth solves this problem completely.]

These nutrients are available in such microscopic dosages that they are rapidly and easily absorbed into the human cellular system, and thereby act as *biological response modifiers*—i.e., they literally help the body modify its ability to absorb larger dosages of nutrients from natural food sources.

No other product we know of today can do this. The micronutrients supplied in Natur-Earth literally "guide" your system in the proper absorption of nutrients from foods, and thereby dramatically increase your body's ability to grow and heal itself. By taking Natur-Earth, along with maintaining a healthy daily diet, your body will have all the nutritional support necessary for cellular repair and growth, thereby enabling it to be more effective in warding off illness and disease.

The SBOs in Natur-Earth are not permanent residents of the intestines. They are there temporarily during therapy and will remain on an active basis for about forty-eight hours if the product is no longer taken. Best results are received when taken every day, as they will colonize on the intestinal wall, doubling themselves every twenty minutes. The SBOs grow very fast and will eat away the attachment sites of candida, hardened mucus, and wastes that are stuck to the intestinal wall, and within pockets or diverticuli found within the colon. Not only do SBOs destroy candida from the inside out, but cause large pieces of it to fall away from the wall of the intestine, thereby quickening its removal.

Observing the results of using Natur-Earth for twelve years, it was shown to be more effective in removing candida, molds, fungus, and negative microorganisms from the body than any other nutritional supplement. The ability for SBOs to grow at a rapid pace and literally devour and destroy a yeast infection throughout the entire body makes this product indispensable for the permanent removal of a candida condition. However, the complimentary ability to encourage immuno-responsive T-cells, anti-bodies, and alpha-interferon to massively accumulate within the systems of the body allows systemic candida that may be in the blood, organs, brain, and tissues to also be neutralized and removed. This again is a remarkable accomplishment when you consider there is little available in systemic remedies for candida.

"The soil-based microorganisms in Natur-Earth are thoroughbreds. Peter Smith discovered the original organism, bred and groomed them, so to speak, and eliminated from them any undesirable elements. When you take a capsule of Natur-Earth, you are taking a thoroughbred selection—highly selected colonies of beneficial soil-based organisms. Peter Smith bred these organisms to perfection,

where the production of undesirable elements is zero—
absolutely zero! That's why I call him a genius."

—Dr. Peter Rothschild

A Major New Weapon Against Viruses, Candida, Allergies

by Dr. Robert W. Bradford, President
Bradford Research Institute

⇒ —— ⇐

*D*ioxychlor®, one of a class of inorganic oxidants, has been found useful against the three major classes of infective agents —virus, bacteria, and fungi—and to have tremendous potential use in such refractory conditions as Acquired Immune Deficiency Syndrome (AIDS). It is also extremely effective against an impressive array of viral, bacterial, and fungal infections, including demonstrated inhibition of *Candida albicans*.

University research has indicated the in vitro effectiveness of Dioxychlor—the premier inorganic oxidant—against the putative "AIDS virus" (HTLV-III/HIV), hepatitis-B, Epstein-Barr virus, cytomegalovirus, polio, and other viral strains. Ongoing in vivo research by the Mexican division of the Bradford Research Institute has confirmed substantial effectiveness against candida, Epstein-Barr, and conditions related to AIDS and AIDS-Related Complex (ARC), Universal Reactor Syndrome (URS), and many lesser conditions.

At the same time, the use of Dioxychlor and the development of specialized microscopy have helped establish what we may call

85

"the pleomorphic foundation of environmental illness." For it has been with the advent of the 7000X phase-contrast video-enhanced computerized imaging system that the systemic invasion of such substances as candida, mycoplasmas, and pleomorphic or "L-forms" (as observed in the blood) may be established. Such microscopy also provides a tool with which to observe the elimination of fungi and bacteria and—with confirmatory electron microscopy—the elimination of viruses. This new dimension in microscopic observation allows the detection of the so-called "L-forms" (pleomorphic forms) which have long puzzled science. The explosive overgrowth of the latter in the body is now being recognized as a virtual market for allergies, sensitivities, and immune depression.

Research on Dioxychlor and its effects is in alignment with the concept of oxidology—the study of reactive oxygen toxic species (ROTS) and their metabolism in health and disease—as enunciated by the Bradford Institute last year. Such research also places Dioxychlor as the major oxidant, of demonstrated effectiveness superior to hydrogen peroxide and ozone, both of which—as indicated below—may be seen as double-edged-sword oxidative therapies.

UNIVERSAL REACTIVE SYNDROME

The institute continues to find evidence that environmental disease—particularly the multiple-sensitivity condition generally denominated "universal reactor syndrome" (URS) almost always characterized by systemic candida and multiple allergies and sensitivities with increasing autoimmune disorders—is to a large extent iatrogenic in nature.

This is because one of the mechanisms that generate so-called "L-forms" is the use of antibiotics, particularly such broad-based spectrum ones as tetracycline, so that the short-term relief of infection provided by such agents is countered by a possible long-term negative: that is, the antibiotics may not be actually killing target bacteria but converting them to pleomorphic forms which may not only be reactivated at a later date but continue to produce toxins and lead to URS. The conversion of bacteria to such L-forms may thus provide relief of symptoms—but at the same time set the stage for later pathology.

Our continuing research indicates that there are two types of pleomorphic forms—reversible and irreversible. One of the primary mechanisms in activating reversible L-forms is the classic oxidative generation response, as in inflammation, antibody-antigen activity, the influenza viruses, and physical and psychological stress.

A classic example is the URS patient—an environmentally ill individual who may be sensitive to everything from hydrocarbons, pesticides and paint, to a wide spectrum of foods. In reality these sensitivities are initiating systemic ROTS ("free radical") substances which in turn activate pleomorphic forms and trigger a clinical crisis reaction which may be far more acute than the sensitivity which set it off.

The above problem is exacerbated by toxins produced by pleomorphic forms, which in turn inhibit the "mixed-function oxidase system," an enzyme complex responsible for detoxifying environmental chemicals, be they organic or inorganic. If the mixed-function oxidase system is blocked or seriously impaired, it leaves the body defenseless against such substances as environmental chemicals.

Indeed, a vicious cycle is set up along these lines.

Step One: Long-term (or even high-concentration, short-term) abuse of antibiotics, contraception pills, corticosteroids, "recreational" drugs, metal toxicity, etc., leads to a general lowering of the immune system.

Step Two: The general lowering of natural immunity leads to a proliferation of microbial infections which in turn are treated by more antibiotics and other drugs.

Step Three: As such infections are treated by antibiotic drugs, microbes convert to, and thus generate, pleomorphic forms. These relatively non-antigenic pleomorphic forms ("cell wall-deficient forms") essentially escape immune surveillance, are resistant to antibiotics, and are capable of existing in all tissues including blood.

Step Four: These new structures in turn produce toxins which, among other things, inhibit the mixed-function oxidase system, the body's primary defense against environmental chemicals.

Step Five: The patient, now essentially defenseless against such chemicals, some of them carcinogenic, becomes hypersensitive to them. These new invaders further depress the immune system.

The result of this five-step biochemical process is the Universal Reactor Syndrome—a situation in which patients increasingly become sensitive to virtually everything in their environment, ranging from actual industrial chemicals to simple foods, and spanning the gamut from reactions to temperature and fluids to the clothing they wear or the sheets on which they sleep. URS becomes a traumatized daily struggle in which an already depressed immune system is constantly turning against itself. The result may be lethal in many cases, but even when not lethal is an unrelenting daily torture.

THE BREAKTHROUGH OF DIOXYCHLOR

Dioxychlor represents a major breakthrough in the eradication of the pleomorphic or "L-forms" whose proliferation is so key to the development of URS. And the improved microscopy allows for the detection of such items in the scenario as system-wide L-forms and mycoplasmas.

Continuing clinical research at Bradford Research Institute, Mexico, has indicated a dramatic reduction in the reactions to all sensitivities through the elimination of systemic pleomorphic forms with Dioxychlor. We have been able not only to reverse URS clinically but—at least in terms of preliminary research—to have an equally impressive response in amyotrophic lateral sclerosis (ALS). This early research suggests a close tie between the symptomatology of ALS and L-form concentrations.

(In many URS patients we also find a significant infection of mycoplasmas—the smallest of the living microorganisms—which are cell wall-deficient structures ranging in diameter from .1 to .5 microns and characterized by a void in the center. The membranes of these forms have receptors for specific human tissues and are prodigious producers of hydrogen peroxide. There are numerous species of mycoplasmas and many are named after the pathologies with which they are associated—for example, pulmonary, neurological, and arthritis mycoplasmas. Mycoplasmas have been destroyed in vivo by Dioxychlor, a fact which may in part account for the dramatic decrease in symptoms of the Universal Reactor Syndrome.

In vitro research indicates the destruction of pseudomonas and the earlier stated viruses within seconds and at low concentrations. *Candida albicans* and Epstein-Barr in vitro tests indicated destruction of the offending structures within seconds at a level of .75 parts per million. Current clinical research suggests such activity is duplicated in vivo.

The Background

Bradford Research Institute, noting that the natural mechanism of action of white blood cells in killing infectious agents is the production of highly active forms of oxygen—namely, the ROTS family—has further described certain inorganic oxidants which also provide active oxygen and mimic the natural activity of white blood cells. These substances include various halogens (chlorine, bromine, iodine) which act as carriers of an active form of oxygen which is later released. For various reasons related to low toxicity, Dioxychlor is the preferred member of this group to be used clinically. Indeed, the potency of the bound oxygen is demonstrated by realizing that Dioxychlor is highly effective at concentrations less than 1 part per million (ppm) that permit it to be used homeopathically.

The use of Dioxychlor as a substance dates back to World War I, when it was used by the Western powers to save the lives of soldiers with infections, particularly gangrene. It has since been found to have a multiplicity of uses which, at first glance, seem unrelated and with no apparent biochemical explanation.

In terms of fungicide use, it is noted that one antifungal agent in common use (nystatin) leads, with prolonged usage, to the development of resistance to the drug and continued symptoms. The mechanism of action of Dioxychlor is related to biochemical processes within the fungus which are so basic to survival that resistance is impossible; as a result, no new resistant strains develop from the use of Dioxychlor, unlike with other fungicides.

Dioxychlor is an inorganic compound composed of chlorine and two atoms of nascent oxygen covalently bonded. It is the chemical property of Dioxychlor which makes possible the release of nascent oxygen upon decomposition during its action as an oxidizing agent, leaving a non-toxic chloride residue. Certain aspects of the cellular immune system (specific white blood cells) utilize other mechanisms in the generation of highly reactive oxygen derivatives for the purpose of combating the invasion of foreign organisms. Without these protective mechanisms provided by the immune system involving oxygen derivatives, the ability to fight environmental chemicals as well as infection is blocked.

The immune system of many persons, particularly the elderly, is deficient in the ability to provide these highly reactive oxygen derivatives so necessary for attacking the great variety of viral, fungal, and bacterial invaders that are continually bombarding the human body. Those who are improperly equipped for fighting these invaders become easy targets for the many diseases they produce, with accompanying and sometimes bizarre symptoms.

The use of Dioxychlor assists the natural protective mechanisms of the body in counteracting these infectious agents which, if not adequately neutralized, will most certainly lead to disease.

Dioxychlor in pure form (anhydrous) is a liquid at 0°C having a deep red color. When mixed with water and at high dilution it is colorless.

Bohr atomic models indicate a "coordinate covalent" bond, but in this bond both electrons are contributed by one of the atoms (chlorine) and none by the other. In the covalent bond one electron is contributed by each of the atoms forming the bond.

When Dioxychlor reacts as an oxidizing agent, the oxygen atom first binds to a single atom (the one being oxidized) and then is dissociated from chlorine. An electron is then given up to chlorine forming the chloride ion. When one realizes that there are 5.3 g of chlorine ion per liter of human plasma, it becomes obvious that the small amount of chloride generated through the use of Dioxychlor is negligible.

Other Cytotoxic Oxidizing Agents Used Clinically

Dioxychlor is not the only oxidizing agent in clinical use. Another agent also providing active oxygen is hydrogen peroxide, which has been used in the treatment of arthritis, cancer, and other metabolic diseases. Hydrogen peroxide is commercially available in low concentrations for the treatment of topical microbial infections.

Ozone is being used both in Europe and at the American Biologics Hospital in Mexico to treat various diseases including cancer, blood coagulation disorders, and liver diseases, among others.

It is a developing precept of oxidology that the success of oxidative therapies depends on the type used, the concentration of the oxidant, and the target of use. For example, hydrogen peroxide may be used effectively as an antiviral sterilizing agent orally and topically. If hydrogen peroxide is used intravenously, great caution should be exercised since, among other things, cancer cells produce prodigious quantities of hydrogen peroxide and the IV administration of this substance may induce cancer to proliferate. This is not true, for example, of either ozone or Dioxychlor.

Ozone is a powerful oxidant which can be used effectively at the right concentration, time, and place—for example, as an intra-tumoral therapy in cancer or in the ozonation of blood to oxidize it and destroy potentially harmful viruses. But any administrative route which increases oxidative processes in the lung is injurious and should be handled with great care; hence the caveat on intravenous ozone administration.

Dioxychlor is currently used as a topical gel ("C2"—complexed with carboners), or as homeopathic drops ("C3"), or as a cryogenically purified intravenous infusion material ("C4").

CYTOXICITY OF DIOXYCHLOR

Proof that Dioxychlor is cytotoxic to bacteria, fungus, and virus clinically is shown by data indicating its effectiveness as a disinfectant (outside the body).

Dioxychlor has been found to inactivate the organism causing Legionnaire's Disease (Legionella pneumophila).

The chemically related compound sodium periodate (NaIO) inhibited the virulence, decreased the respiration of, and increased the sensitivity to, phagocytosis of the common pathogen Listeria monocytogenes.

A germicidal solution was developed containing Dioxychlor at an acid pH (lactic acid). The solution gave complete kill of *Staphylococcus aureus*, pseudomonas, and *Candida albicans* spores within 10 minutes. If used in a ultrasound cleaning device, complete killing occurred in less than five minutes.

The bacterial virus f2 was rapidly inactivated with Dioxychlor. At pH 5-9 only GMP (guanosine monophosphate) reacted, while the amino acids cystine, tryptophan, and tryosine reacted rapidly.

Dioxychlor applied to polio virus separated the RNA from the protein coat (capsid). Dioxychlor reacted with the capsid protein and prevented the absorption, penetration, and normal uncoating of the virus. It also reacted with the viral RNA and impaired the ability of the nucleic acid to act as a template for replication.

QUOTE FROM LEON CHAITOW, N.D., D.O.

_>—<_

Leon Chaitow, N.D., D.O., of London, England, reports that the presence of parasites in many patients can make candidiasis very difficult to treat, and that parasite infestation encourages yeast overgrowth. When treatment results for candidiasis are poor, Dr. Chaitow recommends testing for coincidental parasitic infection. Before treatment for candidiasis, all parasitic infections must first be successfully treated. Researchers believe that candidiasis can become resistant to treatment because of parasites such as Giardia lamblia, amoebas, nematodes, and cestodes.

Parasites can be identified by means of blood, urine, and fecal testing as well as electroacupuncture biofeedback. According to Dr. Chaitow, this method is also useful for revealing how well the body will tolerate any medications which may be prescribed.

To get rid of identified parasites, Dr. Chaitow advises pursuing a comprehensive herbal medicine approach, rather than medication. "In many cases, antiparasitic prescriptive drugs have not proved to be lastingly effective," he points out. "They may diminish symptoms for one or two months, but the symptoms later return with full force." Parasites can be fought with high dosage probiotic substances such as acidophilus, bifidobacteria, and Lactobacillus bulgaricus. Treatment may last from eight to twelve weeks. Dr. Chaitow reports an 80 percent success rate in cases of seriously ill people afflicted with parasites and yeast overgrowth using this method.

—*Alternative Medicine*
compiled by the Burton Goldberg Group

8-WEEK CANDIDA OVERGROWTH ELIMINATION PROGRAM

⋙——⋘

REQUIRED PRODUCTS

Each product is designed to give a specific result. Do not make any substitutions. See page 113 for order form.

Arizona Natural Garlic	*Antifungal and blood purifier*
Caprystatin	*Antifungal for lower bowel, time-released*
Intestinal Cleanser	*Bulking agent to help clean out candida overgrowth*
Coenzyme Q10	*For strengthening the immune system*
DDS Acidophilus	*Restores friendly bacteria (always refrigerate)*
Kaprycidin-A	*Antifungal for stomach and small intestine*
Immuno-Quest	*For strengthening the immune system*
Natur-Earth	*Soil-based organism, antifungal*
Orithrush-D	*Gargle antifungal from mouth to stomach*
Pau D'Arco Tea	*Antifungal and immune builder*
Travacid X	*Digestive aid, time released HCl*
Dioxychlor DC3	*Antifungal/antiviral*
Latero Flora	*Antipathogen/antifungal*
OXY-OXC	*Oxygen therapy*

CANDIDA DIE-OFF REACTIONS

During the 8-week program, it is not uncommon to experience symptoms attributed to the die-off reaction of the candida. These symptoms include feeling tired, spacey, dizzy and apathetic; or you may experience nausea, flu-like symptoms or a goopy sick feeling, muscular aches and pains, skin rashes, headaches, abdominal bloating, rectal itching, irritability, depression, food cravings, and difficulty in sleeping.

You can relieve some of these symptoms by getting plenty of rest at night, exercising, drinking at lease eight glasses of water daily, eating regularly, and keeping snacks available throughout the day. Eating extra protein can also help relieve fatigue.

If you feel overly ill, you should stop the Caprystatin, Kaprycidin-A, and Orithrush-D gargle, but continue the other products until you feel better—usually one or two days. Then continue with the program where you left off.

Colon Therapy Recommendation

You should have one colon cleansing each week or as often as needed during the 8-week program. Bring one quart of Pau D'Arco Tea with you for colon cleansing, which will help to relieve candida die-off symptoms. If you are unable to locate a qualified colon therapist in your area, you should administer frequent enemas.

Colonic... A Gentle Irrigation for Your Colon
Why should I take a colonic?

The colon's main function is the elimination of the body's waste. We experience health and well-being when the colon is clean and normal. When the colon is sluggish, hardened feces lodge in the pockets of the colon walls, resulting in constipation. This hardened matter then obstructs the muscular contractions (peristalsis), reducing the colon's ability to properly evacuate. This waste buildup of many months or years may weigh as much as 15 pounds, causing a distended and abnormally shaped colon. The clogged colon then interferes with final absorption and digestion of food, depriving the body, of necessary nutrients. This results in fermentation and putrefaction of undigested food which creates poisons. These poisons are reabsorbed into the bloodstream and are carried to every part of the body causing a tired and listless feeling. The brain and nervous system become toxic, causing depression and irritability; the lungs create foul breath and stressful breathing; the digestive organs create skin problems and sallow complexion; and the joints may become stiff and painful due to toxic deposits.

Can I be constipated even if I have 1, 2, or 3 bowel movements a day?

Yes. Accumulated wastes, mucous, and gas in the colon may inhibit its natural peristaltic action, resulting in incomplete—though frequent—bowel movements.

What is a colon irrigation?

A colon irrigation is the gradual and gentle introduction of warm, purified water into the colon to help stimulate its natural peristalsis. The colon irrigation, or colonic, tickles the colon walls with water, which helps the colon to release impacted wastes and mucous. Before starting the procedure, the therapist gently inserts into the rectum a sterile, disposable speculum attached to a hose leading to the colonic machine. The client reclines comfortably on his/her back during the course of the treatment, while warm, purified water is slowly administered. After the colon has been sufficiently stimulated, the therapist releases the water pressure. The water and wastes from the colon pass through the hose into the machine's waste drain, and fresh water is again introduced into the colon. The gentle water flow is always under the direct control of the therapist, who repeats the process of fills and releases for 40-50 minutes.

How many times do I need to take a colonic?

Often the waste is so hard and deeply lodged in the colon that a series of colonics may be necessary to sufficiently soften and loosen it. Colonics also stimulate the liver, kidney, and lymph system to dump toxins. The number of treatments varies with each individual and his/her condition. Your therapist can best advise you regarding this.

Are colonics habit-forming?

No. The purpose of cleansing the colon is to allow it to relax and rejuvenate and promote better peristalsis. The colon cannot heal when it is constantly working to get rid of accumulated wastes, gases, and poisons.

Won't colonics damage the normal intestinal flora?

Accumulation of encrusted feces in the colon makes it impossible for the glands to produce the necessary intestinal flora, resulting in increased constipation. Cleansing the colon helps bring the acid-alkaline ratio back into balance, allowing friendly bacteria to thrive, while inhibiting disease-causing organisms. You can assist the body in this process by orally taking acidophilus to reintroduce friendly bacteria into the colon.

DIETARY INSTRUCTIONS

Foods Not Allowed

Beverages: Alcoholic products such as beer, wine, champagne, saki, hard liquor, and liqueurs. Fruit juices, sodas, and other beverages containing natural or artificial sweeteners. All carbonated beverages.

Sugar Products: Simple sugars such as sucrose, maltose, dextrose, galactose, and fructose. Refined sugars (junk sugars) such as white, brown, and raw sugar. Syrups such as molasses, sorghum, maple syrup, and honey. Sugar foods such as candy, chocolate, cakes, pies, cookies, ice cream, sherbet, and any foods with artificial sweeteners.

Fruits: Fresh, dried, frozen, and canned fruits.

Yeast Products: Bread, crackers, brewer's yeast, natural B vitamins, and any products with yeast added (examine labels for vitamin and mineral yeast-based ingredients).

Fermented and Mold Foods: Cheeses, cultured dairy products, buttermilk, sour cream, mushrooms, cider, malts, tofu, soy sauce, miso, pickled foods, vinegar, mustard, catsup, relish, and other condiments made with vinegar.

Peanuts: Peanut butter and peanut products.

Hard Fats: Fats that stay solid at room temperature such as margarine, shortening, and hydrogenated oils.

Processed Meats: Meats and fish that are cured, dried, breaded, pickled, or smoked, such as ham, bacon, corned beef, pastrami, salami, hot dogs, lunch meats, and sausages.

Refined Foods: White flour and white rice.

Tubers: Sweet potatoes, white potatoes, and yams.

Foods Allowed

Beverages: Water (preferably purified), water flavored with lemon juice, herbal teas (no caffeine), decaffeinated beverages, Pero or other grain beverages, and almond milk.

Breakfast Foods: Unsweetened hot cereal, 7-grain, rice flakes, oatmeal, and oat bran.

Carbohydrates: Almonds, sunflower seeds, pumpkin seeds, and Brazil nuts, but no other kinds of nuts or seeds. Puffed rice cakes, legumes, beans, peas, lentils, corn, buckwheat, soybeans, soya products, all grains, millet, and brown rice. Any of these may be ground or combined to make recipes such as noodles, crackers, and breads, as long as no yeast or sugar is added.

Protein: Preferably chicken and fish; however, lean beef, lamb, and veal are acceptable. Moderate use of eggs.

Vegetables: All kinds of cooked and raw vegetables. Frozen vegetables are acceptable, but check labels to be sure they do not contain sugar, vinegar, or additives.

Dairy: Moderate amounts of plain low-fat yogurt, low-fat milk and butter, preferably unsalted raw butter.

Condiments: Spices, herbs, and sea salt. Dressings made without vinegar such as oil and lemon juice or homemade mayonnaise.

Oils: Moderate use of cold-pressed olive oil (refrigerate), sesame oil, almond oil, and tahini.

8-Week Candida Overgrowth Elimination Program Schedule & Dosage

Week One

Date Started: _____ Date Completed: _____

Natur-Earth	*2 upon arising with water only*	⎫
Latero Flora	*2 upon arising with water only*	
DDS Acidophilus	*2 upon arising with water only*	Take these 5 products at the same time
Travacid X	*1 upon arising with water only*	
OXY-OXC	*4 upon arising with water only*	⎭

Dioxychlor DC3 *10 drops under tongue twice daily; hold for 3 minutes, then swallow*

Travacid X	*1 before lunch and dinner*	⎫
Caprystatin	*1 twice daily before meals*	
Coenzyme Q10	*1 twice daily before meals*	Take these 6 products at the same time before meals
Arizona Natural Garlic	*3 twice daily before meals*	
Intestinal Cleanser	*2 twice daily before meals*	
Immuno-Quest	*2 twice daily before meals*	⎭

Pau D'Arco Tea *No more than 6 oz. daily*

Directions: Add 1 heaping tablespoon Pau D'Arco Tea to 4 cups boiling water. Simmer 20 minutes. Strain and refrigerate. Drink either hot or cold.

Week Two

Date Started: _____ Date Completed: _____

Take all products as in the first week, with the following change:

Caprystatin *2 twice daily before meals*

Week Three
Date Started: _____ Date Completed: _____
Take all products as in the first week, with the following change:
Caprystatin   *3 twice daily before meals*

Week Four
Date Started: _____ Date Completed: _____
Take all products as in the first week, with the following changes:
Caprystatin   *3 twice daily before meals*
Kaprycidin-A   *1 twice daily before meals*

Week Five
Date Started: _____ Date Completed: _____
Take all products as in the first week, with the following changes:
Latero Flora   *1 upon arising with water only*
Caprystatin   *3 twice daily before meals*
Kaprycidin-A   *2 twice daily before meals*

Week Six
Date Started: _____ Date Completed: _____
Take all products as in the first week, with the following changes:
Latero Flora   *1 upon arising with water only*
Caprystatin   *3 twice daily before meals*
Kaprycidin-A   *3 twice daily before meals*

Week Seven
Date Started: _____ Date Completed: _____
Take all products as in the first week, with the following changes:
Latero Flora   *1 upon arising with water only*
Caprystatin   *3 twice daily before meals*
Kaprycidin-A   *3 twice daily before meals*
Orithrush-D Gargle   *Mix 1 part with 20 parts water (no refrig-*
                           eration necessary); gargle and then swallow
                           one mouthful of this mixture twice daily.

WEEK EIGHT
Date Started: _____ Date Completed: _____
Take all products as in the seventh week.

CONGRATULATIONS!
You have completed the Candida Overgrowth Elimination Program! Now you should continue with the instructions which follow.

POST-PROGRAM MAINTENANCE
1. After completing the 8-week program, discontinue the following products:
Caprystatin, Kaprycidin-A, and Orithrush-D Gargle.
2. You will have some other products remaining after the eighth week. Finish the remainder of the following products as follows:

Intestinal Cleanser	*2 twice daily before meals*
Arizona Natural-Garlic	*3 twice daily before meals*

3. Continue to take the following products for 3 months as follows:

Natur Earth	*2 upon arising with water only*
DDS Acidophilus	*2 upon arising with water only*
Travacid X	*1 upon arising with water only, and 1 before lunch and dinner*
Latero Flora	*1 upon arising with water only*
OXY-OXC	*4 upon arising with water only*
Dioxychlor DC3	*5 drops under tongue twice daily; hold 3 minutes, then swallow*
Coenzyme Q10	*1 twice daily before meals*
Immuno-Quest	*2 twice daily before meals*
Pau D'Arco Tea	*No more than 1 cup daily*

4. Slowly add restricted foods back into your diet. For the first few days, only add fermented foods. For the next few days add sweet foods, such as fruits, juices, and honey. Try to avoid all alcoholic beverages for 30 days.

If you experience a recurrence of symptoms, return to the restricted diet for 30 days and take three Caprystatin twice daily before meals in addition to the products in instruction 3 above.

5. Avoid commercial meats, commercially-raised chicken, and commercial eggs from caged chickens, since they contain antibiotics, stimulants, growth hormones, and pesticides. Your local health food store should have organic meat, organic chicken (such as Rocky Road chicken), and eggs that are free of these chemicals. You can purchase organic beef from Coleman's Beef, 707 East 50th Street, Denver, CO 80216. Choose wisely, ask questions, and don't settle for less than clean, chemical-free food.

6. At some future time due to illness, you may be required to take an antibiotic. After you have completed the full cycle of the medication, take two DDS Acidophilus capsules daily (with water only upon arising) to rebuild your intestinal flora. This will help you avoid any future candida yeast overgrowth.

LETTERS FROM
SATISFIED CLIENTS

⇒——∈

February 6, 1992

Dear Stanley:

Thank you so much for treating my problem. I have not had any more trouble with candida since I took your treatment.

I am so grateful to you for curing my disease.

I have no rash, no allergic reactions to sugar or yeast foods and my energy is back — all thanks to you. I am not taking any nystatin either.

Wishing you all the best,

Carol Heald

June 22, 1994

To whom it may concern:

As a 27-year employee of a major airline, I found myself exposed, through travel to many exotic ports, to a frightening array of parasitic creatures. For 6 years, I found out the full extent of what traditional medicine did not know. I almost accepted as normal the fatigue, infections, antibiotics, allergies, yeast problems and indigestion that I regularly experienced. Finally, a year ago, I visited Stan Weinberger's Healing Within clinic and took the full parasitic treatment. This was followed by the candida program. I now have a major reduction of all the above-mentioned problems, and the progress is continuing. And while certain portions of the program have required strict dietary restrictions and some discipline, the results are without question worth every effort.

Sincerely,
Loni Blissard
Honolulu, Hawaii

March 24, 1995

Dear Stanley:

I am writing this letter to say thank you for your book, *Healing Within: The Complete Guide to Colon Health*, and for what has happened in my life as a result of reading it.

For years, I have been trying to get to the bottom of why I never felt well. In recent years, I have had a lot of aches and pains and an awful time with constipation and gas and being tired. I tried different diets and was diagnosed once for yeast, but nothing ever seemed to work to make me feel better. I have been to M.D.s, Naturopaths, Health Food Stores, had Cytotoxic Testing, etc. I was always full of gas and either constipated or with diarrhea (constipation has been a longstanding problem with me). Also, I had a lot of tension in my neck muscles and shoulders and low back. I had massage treatments for relief and was at the chiropractor a lot, but nothing ever cleared up any of this. I was really at the end of my rope. But at one point, I felt deep down that somehow when my husband and I moved to the Cape, the Lord was going to help me find the solution to all this chronic stuff.

My daughter is an occupational therapist and massage therapist and she suggested that I try acupuncture for the constipation. But first I saw a nutritionist, Marcia Sloane, at the Cape Cod Center for Holistic Medicine. That was the beginning of the great changes in my health/life.

Marcia told me that I had classic candida symptoms and she started me on a program of diet and supplements. Within three days I noticed a change for the better with my gut/digestion. As the months passed, however, the constipation never really got better. Marcia could not understand it, so we tried acupuncture, but it did not help, nor did the Chinese herbs. I asked Marcia if she thought colonics might help. She said it was certainly worth a try, so I had a treatment. Nothing much changed, but I did feel better in my gut initially.

My husband and I then went to England for six months and I had 13 more colonic treatments and all of the aches and pains and muscle tension went away! I was eating a food-combining diet, losing some weight, and having much more energy. The colonic therapist was also muscle testing me, which indicated that the candida was definitely getting better and I did not show any parasites.

When we came home from England, I continued to feel good and was sticking to the diet, and continued the colonics. But when I went back for a check on the yeast, it was still not as good as it should be. It was very defeating to me that the yeast was still there and I just couldn't understand why this thing can't be licked the way other things can be. Why does yeast so easily come back with the slightest going off the diet?

At this point, I asked Connie Jones, who gave me a copy of your book, whether any of her clients had ever tried your Candida Overgrowth Elimination Program. She said they had, and that they had good results. She suggested I call you and order it.

I did call you, and after explaining my situation, you said that you had found that when candida is so insidious, it may not be the underlying problem. That was very interesting, because so many of my other problems had candida as the underlying cause and now I was hearing there could be an underlying cause for the candida! Sort of like layers of an onion... You suggested that I do the Parasite Elimination Program, which I did. I will admit that I was not totally strict with the candida type diet you recommended, but I stuck pretty much to it.

To make a long story short, I was angry for the first few weeks, and my stomach was as hard as a rock. I knew something was going on. I did call you and you said those were normal kinds of reactions because I was ingesting poison, not nutrients. When I went for a colonic, my right side was extremely sore and tender, which it had never been before, and Connie said that was a very good sign because that is where the parasites like to live.

Shortly before I completed the Parasite Elimination Program, I asked the nutritionist to muscle test me for yeast. She did a lot of testing and when she was done, she said, "What have you been doing? There is NO SIGN OF YEAST AT ALL, NOT EVEN A SUBTLE SIGN!"

I cannot tell you how happy I was. Praise the Lord! Then I told her about the Parasite Elimination Program I had been doing and that this might be an answer for others who have chronic yeast. As I said earlier, after we had moved to the Cape, I really felt that somehow the Lord was going to heal me of the constipation and other symptoms. I think that all I have been through and all my searching was with His help and that somehow this experience of mine may help others down the road. What I want to say is a VERY BIG THANK YOU TO YOU, STANLEY, FOR YOUR HELP.

My constipation problem is getting better too, as I still take extra herbs to stay regular, but now that I have started the Oxy-Oxc, I am taking less of them and think that the Oxy-Oxc is helping. Connie had said that part of my problem may be genetic, which is possible, because my mother and sister have the same problem.

In closing, I want to say that it is a whole new life healthwise for me and even mentally, as I am beginning to remember things much more quickly and just have more energy. I exercise every day and stay up later and do more than I have in a long time. God bless you in your work and for getting the word out. I hope all the yeast doctors who are treating people will not discount the parasite connection in all of this, but see it as another cause.

Sincerely and gratefully,

Laura Lee W.
(last name witheld by request)

OUR INTERNAL
MICROBIAL COMMUNITY—
MAINTAINING THE HEALTHY BALANCE

by Nigel Plummer, Ph.D., Microbiology, University of Surrey, United Kingdom

I t is true to say that we are largely unaware of the friendly microbial community which resides on our skin, and inside our respiratory, genito-urinary, and intestinal tracts. This is somewhat surprising given that they outnumber the total of our own tissue cells by 100:1, and make up about 50% of the weight of our feces. Moreover it should be noted that everything we ingest has to pass through the microbial community before we as the host assimilate it.

In general, the normal flora is very beneficial to our health, protecting us from infection by intestinal pathogens, enhancing the absorption of many nutrients, and detoxifying many of the pollutants we come into contact with on a daily basis. In addition to this there is recent scientific evidence that the normal flora is involved in reduction of cholesterol and the prevention of some forms of cancer.

Unfortunately, this delicate balance of the normal flora can be easily upset, and this can result from circumstances as varied as stressful lifestyle through to the use of prescription medicines. Indeed, probably the most common cause of severe disruption of the normal flora is the use of antibiotics.

Broad spectrum antibiotics are known to have a very major effect on both the numbers and types of the microbial population and one consequence of their use is that undesirable bacteria and yeasts often grow to replace the more beneficial types. These undesirable types can persist for months or years and can produce symptoms in the individual ranging from intermittant abdominal pain through diarrhea or constipation. These symptoms can become chronic and are very similar to those seen in Irritable Bowel Syndrome.

A unique new concept of microbial supplementation is now available which tailors the treatment regime to the level of imbalance in the individual, with the result that in all cases the healthy flora is reestablished and then maintained at optimum levels for maximized long-term benefits. No other system or products differentiate the level of need in the individual and so very often have the effect dramatically under-supplying or over-supplying the beneficial bacteria.

The new system works at three levels:

1. Correcting Major Imbalance. This occurs most often following antibiotic therapy, and acute intestinal upset. Much of the normal flora is eradicated and needs to be replaced very rapidly if overgrowth is to be avoided. As such an intensive period of 14 days supplementation with very high numbers (30-50 billion/day) of beneficial bacteria is advised. After this the normal flora is well on the way to becoming established, and a more extended treatment is required to complete the process. This extended treatment is the same as would be advised for minor imbalance. The product used in this category is called **Replete**.

2. Correcting Minor Imbalance. This occurs in people who live with a stressful lifestyle, or who consume excessive alchohol, and also following general illness. To re-establish the correct microbial balance, a period of 6-8 weeks of an intermediate intensity of supplementation is required (4-5 billion/day). Following this period the flora will be in a balanced equilibrium, and the individual will be poised to obtain the long term benefits of this situation. However, this will only be insured if a maintenance level of beneifi-ial bacteria are supplemented on a daily basis to continually "top up" any sporadic instances of minor imbalance which may occur. The product used in this situation is called **HMF Forte**.

3. Maintaining the Healthy Balance. Once balance has been restored by the above regime, it needs to be maintained in order to achieve maximized benefits of the flora and also to help prevent the system giong out of balance again. By taking this level of beneficial bacteria (1 billion) on a daily basis—but only once the balance is already present—then a healthy beneficial flora is ensured. The product used for this is **HMF**.

THREE PHASE INTESTINAL FLORA REBUILDING PROGRAM

Purpose: To prevent the overgrowth of undesirable bacterias and promote repopulation of beneficial bacteria and enhance removal and detoxification of residual antibodies. This Three Phase Program involves a systematic and *sequential use* of the following:

Level 1—Intensive. Product name: *Replete™ with FOS*

Daily dosage: ½ - 1 envelope dissolved in water with a minimum of 30 billion viable microbes per day.

Duration: Every day for 7 - 14 days.

Strains: Strains of Bifidobacteria, Lactobacillus acidophilus and Lactobacillus brevis are administered. They all have the ability to colonize the gastrointestinal tract. Fructooligosaccharides (FOS) is used in conjunction with these cultures.

Benefits: Rapid establishment of the lactobacilli in the upper small intestine, with Bifidobacteria colonizing the ileum and the colon. Relief of abdominal complaints due to microflora imbalance. Crowding out of yeast and other undesirable bacteria.

Note: Replete should be ideally used the day the antibiotic course is over. If excessive gas develops during use of Replete, use ½ envelope in the A.M. and ½ in the P.M. Each envelope contains 30-40 billion organisms plus 13 grams Fructooligosaccharides (FOS).

Level 2—Follow On. Product name: *HMF Forte (in FOS base)*

Daily dosage: 1 capsule daily delivering a minimum total of 4 billion viable microbes.

Duration: Daily for 6 - 8 weeks.

Strains: High levels of L. acidophilus and Bifidobacteria with lower levels of Lactobacillus brevis. FOS is used in conjunction.

Benefits: Gradual shift of microbial population with beneficial bacteria becoming more dominant. Steady decrease in complaints due to minor imbalance in microflora. Completion of this stage should result in flora being healthy and "normal."

Note: The consumption of cooked oatmeal, fruits and vegetables rich in fermentable fiber (bananas, apples, yams, potatoes) provide excellent nourishment for promoting friendly bacteria growth.

Level 3— Maintenance. Product name: *HMF (in FOS base)*

Daily dosage: Minimum total of 1 billion viable microbes.

Duration: Continuous administration.

Strains: Equal numbers of L. acidophilus and Bifidobacteria in a vegetable FOS base.

Benefits: Continuous supplementation leads to long-term benefits of having optimized flora. Maintenance of healthy flora with lowered risk of imbalance occurring.

Additional Supplements

Before Breakfast:

1 teaspoon of *WheyPlex* - A concentrated fraction of whey that contains the nutrients that support our "gut" defenses.

With Breakfast:

1 capsule of *Poly VytaMyns* - Microcoated multiple vitamin-mineral formula with several cofactors.

1 capsule *Trival* - A 5000 year old formula with multiple distinct properties including a toning effect and gastrointestinal defense support.

1 tablet *Livit 2* - Standardized Ayurvedic botanical formula for liver support. Helps promote detoxification of residual antibiotics.

Before Lunch: 1 teaspoon *WheyPlex.*

With Lunch: 2 capsules *Poly VytaMyns,* 1 capsule *Trifal.*

Before Dinner: 1 teaspoon *WheyPlex,* 1 capsule *Trifal*

With Dinner: 2 tablets *Livit 2.*

To obtain the Three Phase Intestinal Rebuilding Program, please see the order form which begins on the following page.

Healing Within Products

PO Box 1013 • Larkspur, CA 94977-1013

Orders only (800) 300-7548 • in Calif. call (415) 454-6677 • Fax (415) 454-6659

Complete 60-Day Candida Overgrowth Elimination Kit (for all body weights)
  Arizona Natural Garlic (1 bottle, 250 capsules each), Kaprycidin-A (2 bottles, 90 capsules each), Caprystatin (4 bottles, 90 tablets each), Latero Flora (2 bottles, 60 capsules each), Coenzyme Q10 (2 bottles, 60 capsules each), Natur-Earth (2 bottles, 90 capsules each), Colon 8 Intest. Cleanser (2 bottles, 120 caplets each), Orithrush-D (1 bottle liquid concentrate), DDS Acidophilus (3 bottles, 100 capsules each), OXY-OXC (2 bottles, 180 capsules each), Dioxychlor DC3 (2 bottles, 1 oz. each), Pau D'Arco Tea (2 boxes, 4 oz. bulk each), Immuno-Quest (2 bottles, 100 capsules each), Travacid X (2 bottles, 100 caplets each). **Total Products: 29 items. $592.00**
  Each Complete Kit Shipping, Handling & Insurance $12.00

Three Phase Intestinal Flora Rebuilding Program (for all body weights)
  Replete (2 bottles, 7 powder sachets each), HMF Forte (2 bottles, 45 capsules each), HMF (2 bottles, 60 capsules each), Livit 2 (2 bottles, 90 tablets each), Whey Plex (2 bottles, 4 oz. powder each), Vyta Myns (2 bottles, 90 capsules each), Trifals, (2 bottles, 90 capsules each). **Total Products 14 Items. $368.00**
  Each Kit Shipping, Handling & Insurance $10.00

Individual Items	Quantity	Price	Total ___
Arizona Natural Garlic (250 capsules) . . . . ____		14.00	_____
Caprystatin (90 tablets). . . . . ____		18.00	_____
Coenzyme Q10 (60 capsules, 30 mg.) . . . . ____		27.00	_____
Colon 8 Intestinal Cleanser (120 caplets). . . . . ____		8.00	_____
DDS Acidophilus (100 capsules) . . . . ____		17.00	_____
Dioxychlor DC3 (1 oz.) . . . . ____		26.00	_____
HMF (60 capsules). . . . . ____		24.00	_____
HMF Forte (45 capsules) . . . . ____		25.00	_____
Immuno-Quest (100 capsules) . . . . ____		20.00	_____
Kaprycidin-A (90 capsules) . . . . ____		18.00	_____
Latero Flora (60 capsules) . . . . ____		26.00	_____
Livit 2 (90 tablets). . . . . ____		27.00	_____
Natur-Earth (90 capsures) (2 for $80.00) . . . . ____		42.50	_____
Orithrush-D (liquid concentrate). . . . . ____		14.00	_____
OXY-OXC (180 capsules) . . . . ____		30.00	_____
OXY-MAG (4 oz. powder) . . . . ____		35.00	_____
Pau D'Arco Tea (4 oz. bulk) . . . . ____		8.00	_____

Individual Items Cont.   Quantity   Price   Total ___

Item	Quantity	Price	Total
Poly VytaMyns (90 capsules)	___	30.00	___
Replete (7 powder sachets)	___	30.00	___
Travacid X (100 tablets)	___	18.00	___
Trifal (90 capsules)	___	23.00	___
WheyPlex (4 oz. powder)	___	24.00	___
Healing Within: The Complete Guide to Colon Health	___	15.95	___
Parasites: An Epidemic in Disguise	___	7.95	___
Candida Albicans: The Quiet Epidemic	___	11.95	___

MINIMUM ORDER $25.00   TOTAL ORDER _____

California residents add 7.5% tax _____

Shipping, Handling & Insurance for:
Complete 60-Day Candida Overgrowth Elimination Kit: $12.00
Three Phase Intestinal Rebuilding Program: $10.00

Shipping , Handling & Insurance for individual items:
$5.00 minimum. Up to $65.00 add $5.00; over $65.00 add 8%. _____
(See next page for detailed Shipping & Product Information)

TOTAL AMOUNT ENCLOSED _____

Fax and telephone orders accepted only with Visa, MasterCard, American Express, or Discovery. Credit card orders and orders paid with bank checks or money orders are shipped the next working day. Orders paid with personal check will be shipped in 10 days. Send personal check payable to Healing Within Products. No C.O.D. Prices subject to change.

Please print clearly:

Name _____ Day Phone (___) _____

Address _____ Evening Phone (___)_____

City_____ State_____ Zip_____

☐ Visa ☐ MasterCard ☐ American Express ☐ Discover

Card # _____

Expiration Date _____ Signature _____

Healing Within Products

PO Box 1013 • Larkspur, CA 94977-1013

Orders only (800) 300-7548 • in Calif. call (415) 454-6677 • Fax (415) 454-6659

SHIPPING & PRODUCT INFORMATION

Call or Fax Your Order: You may call or fax your order only with Visa, MasterCard, American Express or Discover cards. Business hours are 8:00 a.m. to 5:00 p.m. Pacific Standard Time, Monday through Saturday.

MINIMUM ORDER: $25.00 MINIMUM SHIPPING CHG.: $5.00

Shipping Method: Orders are shipped via UPS Ground. For Second Day Blue Label delivery, double the shipping charges. No shipping on Saturdays, Sundays or legal holidays. Visa, Master-Card, postal money orders or bank checks, American Express, and Discover orders are shipped on the next working day. Orders paid with personal checks will be shipped in 10 days.

Alaska & Hawaii Shipments: For shipments to Alaska and Hawaii, double the continental U.S. shipping charge. Orders will be sent by U.S. First Class Mail.

Canada Shipments: For shipments to Canada, double the continental U.S. shipping charge. Orders will be sent by U.S. Air Parcel Post.

Overseas & Foreign Shipments: For overseas surface shipments, triple the shipping charge; allow 6 weeks for delivery. For overseas air orders, add five times the continental U.S. shipping charge. All foreign accounts must send bank certified checks in U.S. dollars; Visa, MasterCard, American Express and Discover credit cards accepted.

Prices: Prices are subject to change without notice.

Returns: Any items you wish to return must have been purchased within the <u>past 30 days</u>. You cannot return opened bottles or bottles with defaced labels. All returns will have a 10% handling charge. All returned checks will be charged a $10.00 fee.

If you are returning products by UPS, send to:
Healing Within Products
84 Berkeley Avenue
San Anselmo, CA 94960.

If you are returning products by U.S. Postal Service, send to:
Healing Within Products
P.O. Box 1013
Larkspur, CA 94977-1013.

Please call (415) 454-6677 to obtain a Return Merchandise Authorization number. Merchandise not accepted without prior authorization.

Product Storage: We suggest storing your supplements in a cool, dry location. The label will specify if refrigeration is required. These products are for nutritional supplementation only. They are not intended for the mitigation, cure, or treatment of any disease or illness. No other use is assumed, implied, intended, or permitted.